"Work That

"To most people, exercise is a four-letter word (and it's not f-u-n-n). They'd rather clean the house or mow the lawn than go to the gym or take a quick spin around the block (and I don't mean in the car). But what many people don't realize is that housework and yard work are actually good examples of moderate physical activity. Whatever activity you choose is a step in the right direction. I'm here to give you the information you need to improve your health and well-being—one step at a time—along with the motivation to stick with it until you've achieved your personal best.

"Think of me as your paperback personal trainer. I've created a fitness program just for you. In addition to designing separate workouts that you can do at home or at the gym, special routines are included, which you can do outdoors with your family, in the office, or while you're traveling. I'll share the tricks of the trade that I've learned from years of training myself and my clients. You can do this—I know you can. You talk the talk, now it's time to walk the walk. LET'S GET REAL!"

—Donna Richardson

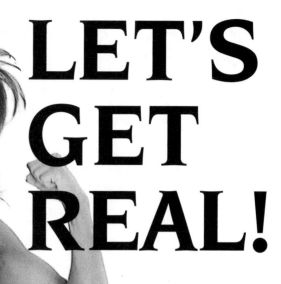

LET'S GET REAL!

Exercise Your Right to a Healthy Body

Donna Richardson

with Lauren David Peden

POCKET BOOKS
New York   London   Toronto
Sydney   Tokyo   Singapore

The author of this book is not a physician and the ideas, procedures, and suggestions in this book are not intended as a substitute for the medical advice of a trained health professional. All matters regarding your health require medical supervision. Consult your physician before adopting the suggestions in this book, as well as about any condition that may require diagnosis or medical attention. The author and publisher disclaim any liability arising directly or indirectly from the use of this book.

An *Original* Publication of POCKET BOOKS

POCKET BOOKS, a division of Simon & Schuster Inc.
1230 Avenue of the Americas, New York, NY 10020

Copyright © 1998 by Donna Richardson
Interior photographs by Norbert Wagner
Interior illustrations © Glen Hanson/Arts Council, Inc.
Portions plate designed by Ron Holt

All rights reserved, including the right to reproduce
this book or portions thereof in any form whatsoever.
For information address Pocket Books, 1230 Avenue
of the Americas, New York, NY 10020

ISBN: 0-671-53883-7

First Pocket Books trade paperback printing March 1998

10 9 8 7 6 5 4 3 2 1

POCKET and colophon are registered trademarks of
Simon & Schuster Inc.

Cover design by Matt Galemmo
Front cover photo by Patrick J. Corley

Text design by Levavi & Levavi

Printed in the U.S.A.

Acknowledgments

❏

I'd like to thank my family, friends, mentors, and colleagues for all their love and support. Special thanks to Kevin Weaver, Sue Carswell, Greer Kessel, Tim Moore, Lorraine Eyerman, and Mary Boyce for all their help and hard work on this project.

Contents

❏

LET'S GET REAL!

Introduction

❑

Fourteen years ago, I took my first aerobics class. The only reason I agreed to participate in such body-bending torture was because my girlfriend Sharon challenged me to do so. Well, honey, let me tell you: *challenged* does not even *begin* to describe how I was feeling. I remember thinking to myself during the middle of the class: "This is pure agony. How much longer will it take for her to realize that we're gasping for breath and sweating our butts off?" We were all ready to wring the instructor's neck, but quite frankly, we were too exhausted. What little energy I had left was steadily diminishing, but I was *determined* to finish. I held out until the bitter end, the moment of glory when the instructor said, "Nice job everyone! Now, let's s-t-r-e-t-c-h."

As it turned out, that class marked my first step toward pursuing a career in the fitness industry. It sparked my passion—some might say my obsession—for exercise, and before long I joined the health club, strutting my stuff in the front row with the best of 'em. Not only did I enjoy these classes, but I found that I was good at them, too, and that aerobics enabled me to combine my twin loves: dance and sports. I had studied dance and physical education at college and had been involved in various sports since I was a kid. These classes eventually led to a part-time gig as an aerobics instructor at a club in Maryland. A year later, I began working at a small aerobics studio in Georgetown, where I was introduced to personal training. I was hooked. I loved the idea of helping folks feel better and look their best. Shortly thereafter, I decided to start my own business, offering personal training and group exercise classes.

I became a personal trainer to some of Washington's movers and shakers, and I taught classes everywhere. I led DonnAerobics classes in churches, schools, hotel ballrooms, corporate offices, community centers, and hospitals. Literally speaking, I taught both the rich and famous and the coupon-clipping folks. I would set up shop wherever there was a need: shaking hands, handing out flyers, and encouraging people to stop by and let me show them how much fun exercise could be. I put up notices in store windows, on bulletin boards—even on lampposts by the side of the road. I was addicted to aerobics, and I wanted to spread the word!

It took a few years of hard work and sweat equity before my business began to turn a profit, but I wasn't in it for the money; I was in it to show people how great it felt to be healthy. I wanted to make exercise accessible to everyone, regardless of their age, shape, gender, race, or fitness level. Eventually I became the owner of my own exercise studio, and if that wasn't enough, I also competed in aerobic competitions all over the world. As I began to make a name for myself in the industry, it was only a short leap—or should I say a short "step-step-clap-turn"—to the wonderful world of cohosting fitness shows on ESPN and to costarring in exercise videos (including Buns of Steel Platinum, Nike Total Body Conditioning and my own series, DonnaMite).

These days, I teach fitness to folks all over the world, and I work as a volunteer fitness consultant to the Boys & Girls Club of America, as well as other children's organizations. I love working with kids, and the experience I've had with them has been gratifying. When I work with those who are less fortunate than I am, it makes me so much more appreciative and thankful for what I have. And believe me, I'm a very happy camper. Additionally, I spend six months out of the year on the road lecturing and conducting seminars, and working as a Nike-sponsored athlete and spokesperson. (By the way, did I mention that my Nike signature shoe, the Donna Richardson Air Max Mundo, came out last year? Not bad, huh?!!)

For me, though, being in the spotlight is only the means to an end. What I really like most about my job—even more than traveling around the world and having my own signature shoe—is that I get to teach people how to lead positive, healthy lives. For Miss Donna (that's the nickname given to me by the kids at the Boys & Girls Club), helping people is what it's all about. I feel the true definition of success is making a difference in people's lives.

I believe that good health is the most precious gift that we can give to ourselves. Many of us treat our health as if it's something we can easily bottle and preserve. *Not!* We must all learn to take responsibility for ourselves by making a commitment to improve the quality of our lives. When you think about it, an investment in your health is an investment in your future.

Ironically, while I travel around the world motivating people to exercise their right to a healthy body, I've discovered that my biggest challenge is within my own family back in Maryland. I don't want to suffer the heart attacks that killed my grandparents, or the strokes that my dad has endured. When I attend a family gathering, I sometimes get depressed because many of my family members are living statistics (at least at this point) for obesity, high blood pressure, diabetes, and heart disease.

I think it's time to stop taking our health for granted and to get up and get moving. Let's get real! It's time to throw away the fad diets, the gimmicks, and the gizmos and restore our faith in ourselves by improving our health and our sense of well-being once and for all. I've been working in the fitness industry for fourteen years now, and there's not a week that goes by when I don't hear about some new, no-effort "miracle" solution that promises to melt away pounds, leaving you with a washboard stomach or killer biceps—without doing a single sit-up or push-up. I don't think so! I'm telling you straight up: *when it comes to fitness and nutrition, there are no miracles.* There's no such thing as a quick fix. Anyone who says otherwise is peddling false dreams and empty promises.

The truth will be our salvation. Facing the truth is sometimes difficult. But when we're honest with ourselves, we're empowered—fear goes right out the window. And the truth about wellness is: it does take time and effort. But the payback that you get from working out and eating healthily is a thousand times greater than the effort you put into it. Fitness is a way of life. It's a lifestyle for a lifetime. I'm not interested in helping you drop twenty pounds in twenty days, because you'll only gain it back again. Forget about killer fitness programs that leave no time for anything else, or giving up the foods you love, or making any other unrealistic lifestyle changes. These are short-term solutions to a long-term problem. They're doomed to fail—and doomed to make you feel like a failure.

What I'm proposing is a moderate, sensible approach to food and fitness that will improve your well-being as well as your waistline. There are no miracles here. However, if you take things slowly, day by day, and make a real effort to incorporate some of my suggestions into your life, you will see a definite, noticeable improvement in the way that you feel and in the way that you look.

You should want to take better care of yourself, not just for today or tomorrow—but forever. This book is designed to help you, but there's one important thing to remember: I can't help you unless you're willing to help yourself. The information in this book will work for you only if *you're* willing to work it. I want to help you break old unhealthy habits and establish healthy new ones.

What I'm offering is the program of a lifetime—literally. If you want to improve the quality of your life, you've got to make physical activity and eating well a full-time habit, not a part-time hobby. As Kenneth Cooper, "the father of aerobics," says, "Good health isn't a destination, it's a journey." One nice thing about shaping your life is that when you start making real progress, it becomes easier and easier until there's just no stopping you. You'll soon be on the move and in the groove!

I say we get down to the nitty-gritty and go back to what I call "Miss Donna's Basics": being active, eating healthy, staying upbeat, and striving to be the best you can be. You've heard the saying "You control your destiny"; starting right now, it's time to put those words into action. I'm here to help you shape up your mind and your body. Believe it—believe in *yourself*—and let's get real together!

1

Let's Get Movin'

If I told you the only way you could have a healthy lifestyle is by jogging five miles a day, doing two hundred crunches, a hundred leg lifts, or eating nothing but egg whites and tuna out of the can, you'd probably close this book right now and never open it again. I wouldn't blame you either. That's why I'd rather concentrate on telling you how you can feel good, look great, and have more energy by making a few minor—and very reasonable—lifestyle changes. Are you still with me? Good. Whether your goal is to run a marathon or walk up a flight of stairs without feeling like you need CPR, a well-designed fitness program like Miss Donna's Basics will help you improve your overall wellness and say good-bye to those love handles once and for all. (By the way, let's call them what they really are: handfuls of fat hanging out in the wrong area. Love's got nothing to do with it!)

I don't know if you've heard the news, but last year, the surgeon general's office released a report that basically confirmed what most of us already suspected: a sedentary lifestyle is hazardous to your health. Did you know that at least 300,000 deaths occur each year due to physically inactive lifestyles and unhealthy diets? Think about it: almost *half a million* people die unnecessarily each and every year. And all because some folks just can't get motivated enough to ease on out of the La-Z-Boy and ease on into their gym clothes. True, gettin' dressed for the cause is only half of it—then you've gotta work that body. Let's start by spending as much time in our sneakers as we do in that recliner. After all, some of us pay almost as much for our sneakers as we do for our furniture—so why no give them equal time?

But working out is only half the story: the best method for reducing your body fat is combining exercise *and* good nutrition. Research has shown that exercise alone is not the answer. What we eat is often the biggest problem. That's why I've included a couple of nutrition chapters in this book, because you need to use both components if your goal is to lose weight.

What I hope to show you is how getting your buns into gear can help you get fit and stay fit. After all, if you can find the time to tune in to the *Today* show or *Nick at Nite*, you can surely set aside thirty minutes a few times a week to improve your bod . . . I mean *health*. If you're really pressed for time, you can even exercise *while* you watch your favorite TV shows or listen to the radio. Hey, you're talking to someone who's done many crunches and push-ups in front of *Oprah*.

Changing your life to make time for fitness reminds me of the scene in *The Empire Strikes Back* when Yoda is teaching Luke Skywalker how to become a Jedi knight. Luke's spaceship has just sunk into a swamp, and his only hope is to try to pull it out by using "The Force." Luke turns to Yoda and says "Okay, I'll give it a try." Yoda replies "No! There is no try, only do or don't." (Yoda would have made a *great* personal trainer.)

To most people, exercise is a four-letter word (and it's *not f-u-n-n*). They'd rather clean the house or mow the lawn than go to the gym or take a quick spin around the block (and I don't mean in the car). But what many people don't realize is that housework and yardwork are actually good examples of moderate physical activity. Whatever activity you choose to do is a step in the right direction towards getting fit. I'm here to give you the information you need to improve your health and well-being—one step at a time—along with the motivation to stick with it until you've achieved your personal best.

Think of me as your paperback personal trainer. I've created a fitness program just for you. In addition to designing separate workouts that you can do at home or at the gym, special routines are included that can be done outdoors with your family, in the office, or while you're traveling. I'll also share some tricks of the trade that I've learned from years of training myself and my clients. You can do this—I know you can. But if you talk the talk, you've gotta walk the walk. To quote my favorite sponsor: *just do it*.

A *special note*: Those of you who are pregnant, disabled, clinically overweight, or over age sixty-five and just starting to exercise for the first time, should check out the info in chapter 5 before beginning my GetFit Program.

Health versus Fitness

When I say the word *exercise*, most people immediately think of lifting heavy weights or running long distances. But there's more to exercise than being able to bench-press 150 pounds or run a six-minute mile. There are actually two types of physical activity that you can do: one to improve your health, and one to make you more fit.

Physical activities that enhance your health include anything that gets you up and moving so that your heart pumps faster. Each of us performs some form of physical activity as a part of our daily lives, from walking around the office to chasing after a rambunctious toddler. Some of the major benefits of moderate physical activity include:

- ◆ Improved functioning of the heart and lungs
- ◆ Firmer, well-toned muscles
- ◆ Reduced body fat
- ◆ Prevention of bone loss (osteoporosis)
- ◆ Lower cholesterol and blood pressure
- ◆ Increased self-esteem
- ◆ Less fatigue, increased energy levels
- ◆ Better mood, reduced anxiety and depression
- ◆ Improved mental cognition
- ◆ Increased life expectancy
- ◆ Improved sleep
- ◆ Improved immune system

Physical activity—the kind that makes you *fit*—follows a more structured program of higher-intensity activities. This form of exercise helps develop the four major components of fitness: aerobics, strength training, flexibility, and body composition.

Probably the most well-known form of exercise is what we in the fitness biz call "cardiorespiratory endurance" (known to mere mortals as aerobics). Aerobic exercise includes physical activities such as walking, swimming, bicycling, and in-line skating. These activities help your heart and lungs to function better. Aerobic exercise is performed by using the large muscles in your body continuously over an extended period of time. For example, swimming a half mile in a pool requires that you use your legs and arms to keep up a steady pace. Therefore, it's aerobic. To perform any aerobic activity, you need a constant supply of oxygen for your body to work. This is what the word *aerobic* means: "with oxygen."

Strength training, on the other hand, is anaerobic, which means "without oxygen." With weight lifting, the goal is to increase the force that the muscles in your body can generate. Lifting heavy boxes, bags of groceries, or a child—all these activities place a premium on muscular strength. Strength training usually requires that you lift reasonably heavy amounts of weight to get stronger. Since we naturally lose strength as we get older, weight training is a critical part of any workout.

Muscle strength is different from muscle endurance. Muscular endurance requires lifting lighter weights to train the muscles of the body to support you throughout a long day. There are some muscles that are considered to be mainly "endurance" muscles because of the functions they perform. For example, the muscles in your lower back and abdominal area (which help support your spine) need to have the strength to support you as you go about your daily business. That support helps prevent back pain and improve your posture. And we all want to stand tall and proud, right?

Flexibility indicates just how supple or tight your muscles are. If they're tight, you won't be able to move your arms and legs easily, making the activities you perform awkward and sometimes even painful (ouch!). To improve your flexibility, you need to stretch your entire body regularly. This will help prevent injuries and relieve life's little aches and pains. One thing that I've learned over the years as an athlete and a trainer is that having a strong, flexible body is the key to ultimate performance in life, whether you're on the playing field or in the boardroom.

The final important ingredient of fitness is body composition—or the ratio of your lean body weight (bones, muscles, and water) to fat. Research shows that people who are overweight tend to have more health problems and a shorter life span than people who are closer to their ideal weight. The great thing about knowing your body composition is that you'll know the percentage of fat in your body. (Like we all *really* want to know that?!!) On a serious note, though, most of us rely on the scale to tell us whether our program is working, but that's really not a good way to measure your fitness success. The scale can tell you only your body weight, not how much fat you have on your body. (And that's an important distinction to make, because muscle is denser and weighs more than fat, even though it makes you *look* fitter. So pump it up!)

Many of my clients ask me about the height and weight charts that some insurance companies use to determine whether or not people are healthy. I've known people who would be considered overweight by the standards of height and weight charts, but when they had a body composition assessment, such as an underwater weighing, their percentage of body fat was low. If your goal is to slim down and shape up, I'd advise you to get a body composition assessment. (I'll give you more info on this a little later.)

Guidelines on Moderate Physical Activity

Most people think of fitness as an all-or-nothing proposition: "If I can't get myself motivated enough to run five miles every day, then I'll never be successful." When my neighbors recently asked me how they could get in better shape, I told them to start a daily walking program. When I saw them the next day, they apologized because they never made it out the front door. I told them, "No sweat. I know you'll take care of it today." As clichéd as it sounds, I really do believe that today is the first day of the rest of your life. If you couldn't find the time to be physically active yesterday, give it another shot today. *Don't give up.*

The good news is that you don't need to spend hours each day slaving away on the StairMaster to boost your energy level and to improve your health and well-being. By doing just a little moderate activity each day, you'll feel so much better. Soon you'll *want* to work that body every day. (I know you're thinking, "*Right*, Miss Donna... *as if.*" But I'm telling you, when you start to see results, they'll be no stoppin' you. And that's a good thing.)

Another good thing is that you can start slowly and work your way up to thirty minutes of physical activity. Best of all, those thirty minutes could be as simple (and as fun) as a walk around the neighborhood with your honey and the kids, taking Lucky for a run in the park, or going for a hike or bike ride with your friends. Just remember to choose something that turns you on. If you like it, you'll stick with it.

Tips on Getting Started

Whenever you start a fitness program, you need to adopt a new attitude toward exercise. If your goal is to lose weight, you need to understand that it's not gonna happen overnight. It took a while to put on those extra pounds, so realistically, you can't expect to lose them in two weeks. (In other words, if you've gained forty pounds since graduating from high school, don't expect to lose all forty in time for your twentieth reunion the week after next.) Instead, let me help you design a safe, effective, and enjoyable fitness program that you can incorporate into your everyday life—a program that will guarantee results if you stick with it. But before we begin, let's review some of the major fitness-related decisions and think about how to approach them.

◆ Should you exercise alone or work out with others? This is really a matter of personal preference. Some people love to take a long solitary run or walk, using the time to unwind and recharge. Other people view exercise as a time to socialize and prefer group activities like aerobics classes or a communal hike. Experiment to find what works best for you. It could even be a combination of solitary and group activities: cross-country skiing alone one day and taking a yoga class with friends the next.

◆ Where should you work out? Design a convenient fitness program that you can do at home, at work, or at a place close to you. This is an area where I have lots of firsthand experience. I travel constantly, so I've developed a program that lets me get busy anywhere. I can do my routine at home, at the gym, at the office, or on the road. All I need is a pair of sneakers, my jump rope, and my rubber tubing (it's nothing kinky) and I'm good to go.

◆ What about those days when you feel like you barely have time to breathe, let alone work out? Instead of putting exercise on the back burner, make the most of the time you do have. If you've promised to spend an hour with the kids, don't do it sitting in front of the television set. Instead, take them out to play. If you're hammered at work and can't get to the gym for your usual lunchtime workout, close your office door to get in a few crunches or stretches, or wait until you get home and do a little "sumthin' sumthin'." The important thing is to try to make efficient use of the time you have. I like to keep a T-shirt, a pair of shorts and sneakers in my car so that if a meeting gets canceled or I unexpectedly find myself with extra time, I have everything I need for a quick workout.

◆ How often should you work out? Be careful not to overdo it. Take it one step at a time. As we all know, Rome wasn't built in a day. Select low-to-moderate intensity activities that will help you establish lifetime fitness habits. Walking, for instance, is a good beginner's activity, and low-impact or water aerobics are better choices than high-impact activities. The idea is to start slowly and work your way up the fitness ladder. If you try to do too much too soon, you may be overwhelmed and feel like you just can't keep up the pace.

◆ How can you avoid boredom? Instead of following a "cookie cutter" routine day in and day out, mix it up by cross-training. Choose a few different activities and incorporate them into your routine to keeps things lively. Variety is the spice of life—so let's spice up that workout!

◆ So you don't want to drop big bucks to join a health club or buy fancy fitness equipment? Hey, dancing is free. And you can do a lot of other exercises without having to spend a dime. (Ever try hoisting a two-year-old over your head? It's quite a workout.) Use your imagination.

◆ How can you tell if you're making progress? Use goal-setting and record-keeping strategies such as a training log to chart your success. (I've included a fitness/nutrition diary at the back of the book that you can use to keep track of your progress.) If you want an expert's opinion, you might consider hiring a personal trainer to help motivate you and supply some positive feedback. (Many gyms now have trainers on staff who will monitor your progress and help update your routine every few months, at no extra cost.)

Setting S.M.A.R.T. Goals

Beginning any new adventure requires that you set goals at the outset. How else will you know if you've achieved what you set out to do? A simple formula to use when setting goals for your fitness program is the easy-to-remember phrase: "Think S.M.A.R.T." S.M.A.R.T. stands for Specific, Measurable, Attainable, Realistic, and Timed. By including all of these elements into your goal-setting process, your chances for success improve tremendously. Saying, "I'm going to lose weight" is not a S.M.A.R.T. goal. It is not specific enough, not measurable (how much weight?), and not timed. A better thing to say would be, "I am going to lose ten pounds over the next two months by eating less fat and exercising at least three times a week." This is definitely a S.M.A.R.T. goal, since it is specific, measurable, attainable, realistic, and timed. Get it? Got it? Good.

There are a few other things you should consider when setting your fitness goals. When I work with people I always want to set my clients up for success. You need to start off by *not* focusing all your efforts on achieving your ultimate goal, since it may be too much for you to handle. (After all, the biggest obstacle you'll face in the beginning of any fitness program is just getting your butt up and moving.) To help ensure your success, the best thing to do is choose short-term, intermediate, and long-term goals. For short-term goals it's important that you pick several that are relatively easy to achieve. Buying this book and reading it cover to cover is an example of a short-term goal that anyone can achieve. Setting aside some time during the day to do your thirty minutes of moderate activity is also another attainable short-term goal. Each of these goals builds on the next one. For example, having a short-term goal of doing thirty minutes of moderate physical activity a day can lead to an intermediate goal of joining a health club in the next six months. Suddenly, *voilà!* You've achieved your long-term goal of losing fifty pounds over the next year.

Remember: *you can do it.* It's simply a matter of making yourself—and your health—as much of a priority as everything else in your life. I can't promise you that it will always be easy, but with a little planning and preparation, becoming more physically active is definitely doable.

Take it from me: I have an incredibly hectic schedule, and sometimes I feel like I don't have a second to spare. But I make sure to fit in fitness. If that sometimes means running the stairs in my hotel or sneaking in a set of push-ups between meetings, so be it. Taking the time to get my body moving is the best thing I can possibly do for both my physical health and my emotional well-being. Are you getting my drift? Try working out for just a few weeks, and see if you don't find yourself saying, "Girlfriend was *right!*" The time you spend working out will leave you with energy and zest, so you'll actually be able to do your thing, and then some.

2

Let's Get Healthy

I've already told you a little bit about working out to get healthy versus working out to get fit. The basic difference has to do with how hard, how long, and how often you work out: working out to get *healthy* involves doing moderate activities (a little bit of gardening here, a walk in the park there) that will help you live longer, put some pep in your step, and lessen your chances of getting heart disease, cancer, and many other ailments. Working out to get *fit* involves a more structured exercise program (at least twenty minutes of continuous, heart-pumping activity three to five times a week) that will give you the same health-boosting benefits as moderate exercise but will also turn your bod into a lean, mean fit machine. But before you can begin to get fit, you have to get healthy. After all, if you haven't gotten off the couch in a while, there's no way you can expect to suddenly jump up and bike ten miles, or begin pumping iron like there's no tomorrow. You have to learn to walk before you can run. Or even jog, for that matter.

In days gone by, fitness was built in to people's everyday lives, and our ancestors stayed strong and healthy almost by default. During the first half of the twentieth century, most Americans spent long days working the farm (milking cows and plowing fields could be considered pioneer-era aerobics)—and before farming, people had to go out and forage for every single meal. (It's amazing how easy it is to keep your weight down when you're running from a woolly mammoth or chasing

15

down a mastodon for dinner!) Today, of course, we live for convenience. Technology has made our busy lives easier to manage, but it has also robbed us of the built-in activity that was once central to human existence. Before cars were invented, people often walked to their destinations. Likewise, the food our ancestors ate was more likely to come straight from their gardens or farms than from Burger King. There was no such thing as "health food" because it was *all* healthy—they didn't have all those additives and preservatives and Red Dye No. 9! And fast food was something you could whip up in less than three hours, not something you ordered at the drive-through window. When we're hungry these days, we simply make our way down to the supermarket and pick up some prepackaged food, drive to the local Taco Bell, or simply sit in our nice cozy recliner and order takeout (no hassle there!), then eat it while watching our favorite television show.

Given all this convenience, it's no wonder that Americans are growing fatter and less healthy than ever before. You know that old-timer's lament: "When I was your age, I used to walk a mile to school every day, even in the snow"? Well, it's probably true! Unlike great-grandpa, we have to make an *effort* to move our butts, since it's no longer a built-in facet of our daily lives. And when it comes to being active, the thing to remember is that your body is a machine, just like your car. You wouldn't park your car in the garage for two years, never run it, then expect it to perform perfectly the next time you took it out for a spin, would you? Well, the same "move it or lose it" principle is true of your bod. If you want it to run smoothly and last a lifetime, you have to use it on a daily basis, and you have to give it premium fuel in the form of nutritious food.

In the beginning, the key to becoming healthy is to squeeze physical activity into the time you already have, instead of trying to find extra time. It's a lifestyle approach, and it's all about getting maximum benefits in minimum time. You need to sprinkle fitness throughout your day because what matters in terms of health benefits is the total amount of exercise you get during the day—not whether you do it all at once. So if you don't have time to do twenty continuous minutes of activity, try to sneak in five minutes here and ten minutes there. You'll be amazed at how easy it is to fit fitness into your life!

One of the biggest obstacles to getting healthy is a "can't do" attitude. You know how easy it is to find excuses not to exercise. *Let's Get Real!* You're *never* too old, you're *never* too fat, and you're *never* too busy to get busy. People think of these challenges as disabilities, but they're only disabilities if you *allow* them to be. I mean, really, when you get right down to it, we're *all* very busy, and we're *all* maturing—these are just facts of life. Are you gonna let this keep you from looking and feeling your best? I say, no way, José! When it comes to getting and staying fit, it really is mind over matter. Changing your mental outlook is the key to long-term success. Most people set themselves up to fail by taking the "all or nothing" approach, believing that if they can't give it 110%, then it's not worth doing at all. When it comes to physical activity, though, nothing could be further from the truth. Working little bits of activity into your day may not give you a washboard stomach and Schwarzenegger-size biceps, but it *will* make your body function better, and it *will* increase your longevity. You have to start somewhere, right? Trust me on this one: start small, by introducing physical activities into your daily life a little at a time, and you will soon see big health benefits. Being healthy involves doing activities that work for you on a daily basis. I think of successful health-related activites as incorporating the "Three As:" Anytime, Anywhere, Anybody. (A*men!*)

One easy way to get healthy is to spice up the activities you already do with some fitness moves. Remember the movie *Karate Kid*, where the old man made the boy do all kinds of household chores, and then ended up turning them into karate lessons ("Wax On, Wax Off," and "Paint the Fence")? Here are some examples of daily activities that can be turned into moves that can help make you healthier:

- ◆ Overhead shoulder press grocery lift to cabinet
- ◆ Squat and baby curl (squat slightly while lifting junior)
- ◆ Leaf raking torso twist
- ◆ Vacuum push and pull
- ◆ Corner cobweb dusting reach (for flexibility)
- ◆ Broom sweeping twist (for flexibility)

By combining what are known as ADLs, or activities of daily living, with standard exercise moves, you get a more comprehensive workout that will help you function better throughout your day. Be creative! Let your imagination go and think of some other activities that you can do to boost your fitness level. To help you out, here is a list of the basic and advanced ADLs:

> *Transfer activities.* Sitting to standing, including getting up from a chair or climbing into your car.
>
> *Walking activities.* Includes negotiating curbs and stairs, opening doors, and carrying items.
>
> *Light housework.* Dusting, mopping floors, washing dishes.
>
> *Gardening.* Kneeling, raking, digging, watering.
>
> *Shopping.* Pushing a cart, carrying grocery bags, reaching for products on shelves.

Once you've successfully increased the amount of activity in your daily life, you can then move on to a more structured fitness program (the kind that'll build your biceps and whittle your thighs). Adding just a few activities a day will make you feel better, look better, and will help you become healthier. Before long, you'll be ready to move into a full-time fitness groove. For now, though, try to incorporate at least one of the following get-healthy activities into your life each week, until you find that being active is second nature. And even after you adopt a more structured exercise program, you'll still want to keep up your new, active lifestyle. Most people who are successful in losing weight and staying fit have learned to blend both aspects of fitness—everday activities plus a structured workout program—into their life. Here are some activities to help you get up and get moving:

Cleaning the House. This is a great health-boosting activity, and it's something most of us have to do anyway. The next time you need to clean the house, don't look at it as a mundane chore but as a step on the road to a more active lifestyle! Thirty minutes of vaccuming burns about 123 calories for a 150-pound person, and you can get more bang for your fitness buck if you take time to move the furniture and get into

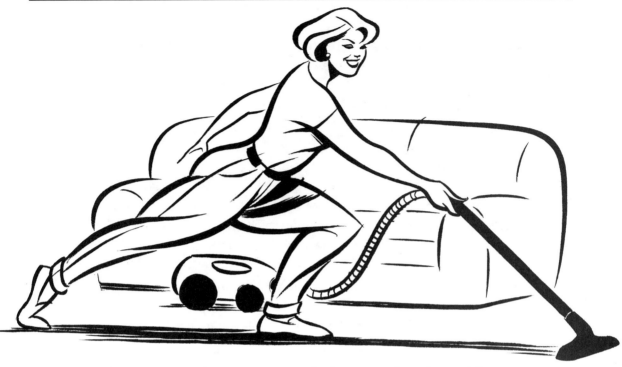

all those nooks and crannies. Instead of just standing there while you vaccum, work in some lunges by taking extra-big steps. Pushing the vaccum back and forth aggressively will get your heart pumpin'.

Dust with gusto and really put some muscle into it! If you're mopping, you can give your arms a workout while you buff that floor to a high shine. You can do the aforementioned Broom Twist to help increase your flexibility (simply rest the broom on your shoulders, drape your arms over it, and twist your upper torso from side to side). Need a little motivation? Pretend you've got folks coming over and you want to pass that Spic and Span test with flying colors. (You know, with everything lookin' nice and shiny.) That oughta do the trick.

Shopping. We all have to eat, so we all have to shop. The next time you hit the grocery store, don't just grab a cart and get right down to business. Instead, take a five-minute walk around the aisles to get your heart pumping. Along the way, you can say hi to your neighbors and scope out the weekly specials. Then, get a cart and fill it with the healthiest food you can find. You get bonus points for maneuvering through the aisles without stopping (use the push-and-grab move, pushing the cart with one hand while reaching for your groceries with the other). When you get home, do the overhead grocery press lift to the cabinet: hold two equal-size cans or jugs at shoulder level, then lift your arms straight overhead and bring the cans together. Do this several times before putting them in the cabinet. (And don't forget to eat something before you shop! I have finished many an ice-cream sandwich before the cashier has even rung me up.)

Watching TV. Sitting in front of the television set doesn't have to be a passive activity. The first thing you can do to make TV viewing more active is to hide the remote and get up to change channels manually (a radical concept, I know, but it will help get your butt in gear). If your television set it just out of arm's reach, use changing channels as an excuse to do a nice looong stretch. You can also do some leg lifts, push-ups, and crunches while watching TV. Oh, and what works for me is doing crunches with my honey. I'm telling you, crunches have never been so stimulating and exciting.

Yardwork. Think a beautiful yard is easy to maintain? No way. One way to help your flowers flourish and increase everyday activity is to throw out those high-tech gardening tools and become a human Weedwacker. Pulling weeds can help strengthen your upper back and arm muscles, and it will certainly get your heart pumping faster. So will thirty minutes of raking leaves, shoveling snow, and turning over the soil to plant new seeds in the garden. (Do the Rake Twist, as mentioned earlier, which will help stretch and tone your back and stomach muscles. Simply stand in one spot and twist your body to gather up all the leaves on the ground around you.) Likewise, when it comes to mowing the lawn, leave the fancy-schmancy riding mower in the shed and use grandpa's old push mower instead. Mowing your lawn the old-fashioned way burns a whopping 420 calories an hour and is a great overall workout. (That's what they tell me, anyway. I have yet to work it out in the yard.)

Washing your car. The next time you need to wash and wax your car, don't go to the automatic car wash—do it yourself and get a miniworkout (to the tune of 315 calories an hour)! Soap the car up methodically using big arm motions, then hose it off while stretching as much as you can. When it comes time to apply the wax, really get into it and use elbow grease to buff the finish to a high shine. When you're done, your ride will look great, and so will you!

Doing laundry. Most of us do the wash once a week, at least. Instead of rushing through the wash-and-dry routine, take a few minutes to make this a more active chore. Do squats while you fold the whites, and work in some stretches while you sort the colors. If your washer-dryer is in the basement and you're feeling really motivated, don't try and carry both loads up the stairs at once. Take one load up, put it away, then come back down and get the second load. This will add a little more physical activity to an everyday chore.

Talking on the phone. The next time you let your fingers do the walking, make sure the rest of your body follows suit. Don't just sit there doing nothing while you chat away—get up and move around. (What do you think cordless phones are for, anyway?) When your friends call, put them on speakerphone and get in some bicep curls or tricep dips (you only need to grunt "uh-huh, you said it, girlfriend" every few minutes to keep up your end of the conversation).

Commuting. Bike to work instead of driving. If you use public transportation, get off the bus or subway a couple of stops early and walk the rest of the way. In the morning, you can use this time to help get yourself revved up to face your workaday challenges; when you're on your way home, a walk will help you unwind and relax.

At work. When you're at the office, use the stairs instead of taking the elevator. Don't spend endless hours in front of the computer screen— it'll fry your brain and give you what some people call the "secretary spread" (I call it butt spread). Instead, make a point of getting up from your desk every hour or two to stretch out and take a brisk stroll around the office. Keep a big glass of water on your desk, and use these breaks as an excuse to fill 'er up!

3

Get Fit

Now that you've started incorporating the ADL's (activities of daily living) into your everyday routine, it's time to get into a more structured program—which means working out for twenty to sixty continuous minutes at least three times a week. Here are Miss Donna's Tips for Getting Started:

1. *Consult your doctor.* Before you begin any fitness program, the first thing you need to do is check in with your doctor. Your doctor should give you a basic exam, which includes checking your heart and lungs, to determe any factors that might limit the types of exercises you can do. This exam usually includes taking your resting heart rate and blood pressure, and having a blood test to determine your cholesterol levels. According to the American College of Sports Medicine (ACSM) Guidelines, a physician should obtain a medical history questionnaire before giving you the go-ahead to break a sweat.

With the information obtained from the questionnaire, you will be classified into one of three categories: apparently healthy; individuals at increased risk; and individuals with known disease. Knowing where you figure in is an important part of developing a safe and effective program. It helps to determine the type of program you should follow and also whether you might need further medical evaluation for more serious problems.

2. *Set realistic goals.* You need to set short-term and long-term goals to ensure that you achieve the results you're looking for. What is it you want to accomplish with your fitness program? Do you want to lose weight? Build muscle? Have more energy and zip? Define realistic goals for yourself, and let me help you design a plan of action to make your dream a reality.

3. *Choose activities you like that will help you reach your goal.* If you're trying to slim down and tone up, there's really no secret to it: you need to do a minimum thirty minutes of aerobic activity at least three to five times a week, and to participate in a two-to-three-times-a-week strength-training program. Both will help you burn fat, add muscle to your body, and crank up your metabolism. Your body will become a continuous fat-burning machine—even when you're at rest. (Now ain't that something?!)

4. *Eat well-balanced foods in moderate portions.* When it comes to getting—and staying—in shape, being active is only half the story. Food is the other half. Exercise will help burn calories and boost your overall metabolism, but if you're consuming more calories than your body needs to function, you won't lose weight. It's that simple. Exercise and diet go hand in hand, and they're equally important.

5. *Be consistent.* That's the only way you're going to get results. Work on achieving your goals each and every day. Make exercise and eating well part of your daily routine. Half the battle is getting started (it takes about twenty-one days to break old habits and establish new ones), but stick with the program, and you'll be slim and trim in no time.

Miss Donna's GetFit Program

The first stage of any fitness program usually lasts about four to six weeks, which is just enough time to start getting your body into better shape. Your heart and lungs become stronger and more efficient at doing their jobs, your muscles get toned, and your energy level increases. Plus, you get into the habit of working out regularly. (After a while, it will become as routine as brushing your teeth. I promise.)

During this phase of your fitness program, you should start slow and build on your level of activity. I can't stress that word enough—go *sloooowww*. Don't take on too much too soon. Otherwise, you may get overwhelmed and feel like you can't keep up. And then you know what happens—you just wanna shout the two words Miss Donna hates to hear: "I Q _ _ T." But I'm not hearing that, honey! You've gotta trust me on this: take things nice and easy, and you'll reach your destination soon enough. (Remember those old Bugs Bunny cartoons where Bugs got himself all lathered up racing the take-his-own-sweet-time tortoise? Remember who always won? Make like the turtle and you'll do just fine.)

Way too many people are devoted to the "no pain, no gain" philosophy of exercise, which is a total fallacy. People who participate in high-intensity exercise tend to have more injuries and higher dropout rates than folks who follow more moderate routines. This is especially true for those of you who are just beginning an exercise program, because you really are starting from scratch. Again, you have to learn to walk before you can run.

Speaking of walking, I think this is a *terrific* way to shape up when you're just starting out—and it's one of my favorite ways to stay fit. But you also have to include the other ingredients of the fitness recipe: strength training and flexibility. Together, they add up to a well-rounded program that will help you get into the groove of your new routine. With Miss Donna's GetFit Program—which includes a walking routine, an at-home and at-the-office strength-training program, and warm-up and cool-down stretches—you'll soon be on your way to a fitter... I mean *fabulous* ... you!

Warm It Up!

The first thing you need to do before exercising is to warm up. The purpose of the warm-up is to elevate your heart rate, warm up your muscles, prepare your body for action, and reduce the risk of injury. You should do a few stretches before exercising, but you can't stretch cold muscles.

To warm up, take a brisk walk or march in place for five minutes. A warm-up helps to increase the temperature of your body, making the muscles more supple. Try stretching a rubber band that you've had in the freezer and you'll see what I mean: it will break if you pull on it.

Once you've warmed up, it's time to stretch it out. (Think of it this way: you don't just gun your car's engine on a cold morning and take off down the highway at sixty miles per hour, do you? No, you let it warm up so it performs better. Your body's no different.) Here are six stretches that will help get your engine going and prep your body for the workout to come. Remember to hold each stretch for five to seven seconds, then you'll be ready to get busy.

Stretching 101

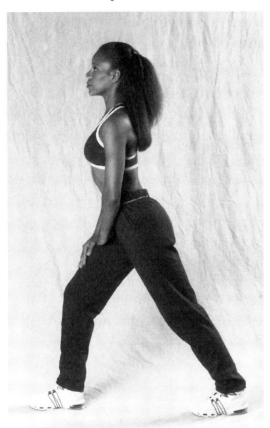

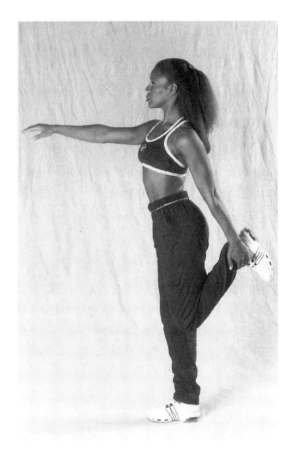

Calf Stretch

Start by standing with your legs about hip width apart, your shoulders and hips square to the front. Lunge forward with your right foot so that your left foot trails straight behind you (right leg bent, left leg straight). Place your hands on top of your right thigh and slowly move your hips forward until you feel a stretch in your calf. (To get a good stretch, keep the heel of your left foot on the floor and the toes of both feet pointed forward.) Switch legs and repeat.

Quadriceps Stretch

Stand with your feet slightly apart, knees soft, and abdominals in. Place your hand on top of your foot and curl your leg up toward your buttocks. To help maintain your balance, extend your arm in front of your body or rest your hand on a wall for support. Gently pull on your foot until you feel the stretch in the front of the thigh. Hold the stretch for five to eight seconds, and return to the starting position. Repeat with the other leg.

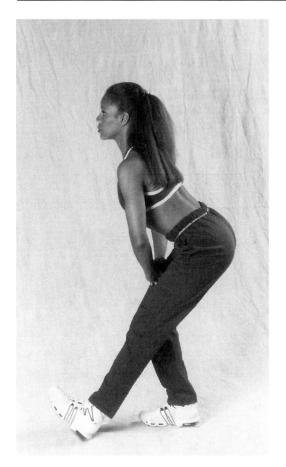

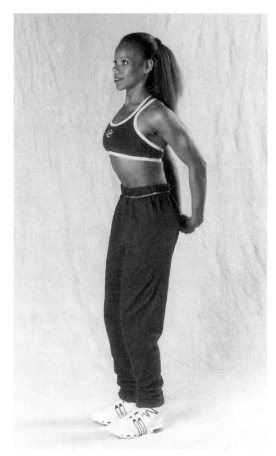

Hamstring Stretch

Stand erect with your feet slightly apart. Extend your left leg forward on the floor, keeping your right knee slightly bent and your back straight. Bend at the waist, lowering your upper torso toward your left thigh. Hold for five to eight seconds. Return to starting position and repeat with right leg.

Shoulder and Chest Stretch

Stand erect with your feet shoulder width apart and your abdominals tucked in. Grasp your hands behind your back, keeping your elbows slightly bent and your shoulders down. Lift your arms slightly away from your body, and focus on opening from the chest as you squeeze your shoulder blades together. Avoid arching your back. Hold for five to eight seconds, then return to starting position.

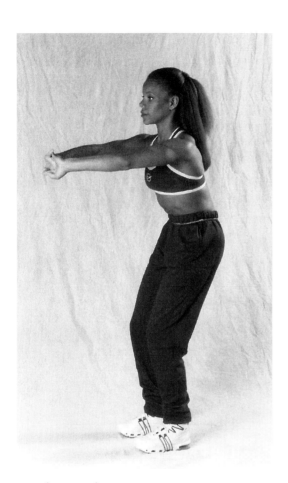

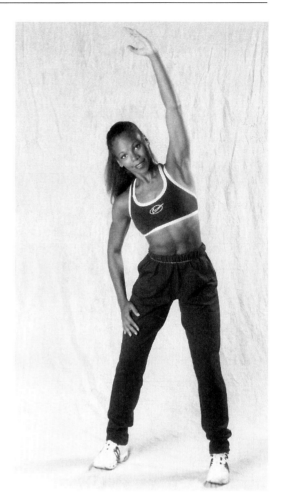

Back Stretch

Start with your feet shoulder width apart and your abs contracted. Grasp your hands together in front of your chest, then press your palms forward. As you lengthen your arms, round your back. Hold for five to eight seconds then return to starting position.

Side Stretch

Stand with your feet shoulder-width apart, your right hand on your right thigh. Extend your left arm overhead and bend slightly at the waist. Hold and repeat on the other side.

WALK IT OFF!

Walking: you can do it anytime, anywhere. You don't need expensive equipment or a fancy gym—walking is free. All you need is a good pair of shoes. It's low impact, burns lots of calories, and strengthens your heart and lungs. No matter what your age, fitness level, shape, or size, walking is good for everyone.

First focus on your posture—walk tall with your abs tightened in to protect your back. Lift your chest and keep your shoulders relaxed with your eyes cast several feet ahead of you. When you walk, practice good technique. Concentrate on rolling from your heel to your toe with each step. This allows your ankle to move through a full range of motion. Also, extend your leg to fully complete your stride, which will help you maintain the proper pace and keep your body correctly aligned.

In order to move at a faster pace—the faster you walk, the more calories you burn—bend your arms at a ninety-degree angle, keep them close to your body, and pump them as you walk. Don't swing them like crazy, just let it flow naturally. (And leave your hand and ankle weights at home because the potential risk for injury just isn't worth the few extra calories they help burn. Walking with weights can place strain on your joints and muscles. Ouch!)

I've designed four different routines—from beginner to advanced—that will help get you in tip-top shape. The nice thing about my program is that you can walk for as little (fifteen minutes) or as long (sixty minutes or more) as you like, regardless of your fitness level. If you're just starting out, begin at the lower level of the program and gradually work up to the high end, using the "10 Percent Rule." It works like this: if you started out walking three times a week for twenty minutes each time (a total of sixty minutes for the week), you would add on a maximum of six minutes to the total time of your workouts. The next week you could spread those six minutes over your three workouts, adding two minutes to each walking session, for a total of twenty-two minutes. As you progress up the fitness ladder, make your walks more challenging by throwing in some hills, increasing your pace, going on an all-day hike, or by incorporating running into your program.

Miss D's Four-Part Walking Program

Time	Distance	Pace
Program 1, First Timers		
Walk 15 minutes	$1/4$ to $1/2$ mile	
20 minutes	$3/4$ mile	
30 minutes	1 to $1^1/2$ miles	
45 minutes	2 to $2^1/2$ miles	
60 minutes	3 to $3^1/2$ miles	20-minute miles
Program 2, Advanced Beginners		
Walk 15 minutes	$1/2$ mile	
20 minutes	1 mile	
30 minutes	$1^1/2$ to 2 miles	
45 minutes	$2^1/2$ to 3 miles	
60 minutes	$3^1/2$ to 4 miles	15- minute miles
Program 3, Intermediate		
Walk 45 to 60 minutes	3 to 4 miles	14-minute or 13-minute miles

◆ Add a hill or incline in the first mile (on a treadmill, increase the incline from 0 to 3 to 4 percent).

◆ Add rolling hills throughout the walk.

◆ Sign up for a 5K walk.

TIME	DISTANCE	PACE

Program 4, Advanced

Walk 60 minutes.   4 to 5 miles   12-minute miles

◆ Walk 4 minutes at a fast pace and 4 minutes at a slower—but still brisk—pace.

◆ Walk intervals of 3 minutes fast and 2 minutes brisk.

◆ Walk intervals of 2 minutes fast and 1 minute brisk.

◆ Go on an all-day (4- to 6-hour) hike in the mountains.

◆ After you can walk at the above pace for 45 minutes, alternate 2-minute jogs with 4-minute walks, and slowly increase the time you jog and decrease the time you walk until you can comfortably run for 20 minutes straight.

Choose a walking program that fits your needs and style, both of which will change over time as you become more fit. Also, it's important to add other aerobic activities into your weekly program to cross-train your muscles and to keep you from getting bored. If walking is your main cardio workout, try adding one or two other activities—such as aerobics, kickboxing, in-line skating, or spinning—to round out your fitness routine.

As you begin to get into your program and start making some progress, always remember the following golden rules:

1. *The 10 Percent Rule.* Increase your mileage no more than 10 percent each week.
2. *The Time Off Rule.* If you take some time off—because you're sick, let's say—start back at a lower level and work your way up again.
3. *The Hard/Easy Rule.* Alternate difficult workouts with a day of rest or an easy workout to allow your muscles to recover. That way, you'll always perform at your peak.

Pump It Up at Home

As I've already mentioned, two of the biggest stumbling blocks for people just beginning an exercise program are time and convenience. Home exercise equipment and fitness videos have become very popular because they overcome these obstacles. To help you out, and save you some money in the process, I've designed a home workout routine using objects in your home. It's time to get you moving!

To start your at-home program, you'll need a couple of bottles of water, or two- to five-pound dumbbells, if you have them. Make sure to lift the weights using slow, controlled movements. Do the following strengthening exercises for just fifteen minutes a day, twice a week, and you'll definitely start to get hooked on the fitness habit. If you are just starting a fitness program or getting back into the swing of things, begin by doing each component of the exercise separately. As you begin to make progress, combine both exercises as prescribed here. Do one set of eight to twelve reps for each exercise. (And check out my cousin Monique in the at-home workout photos. I've got my whole family doing the fitness thang!)

Step Up and Bicep Curl (works the thighs, buttocks, and front of the arms)

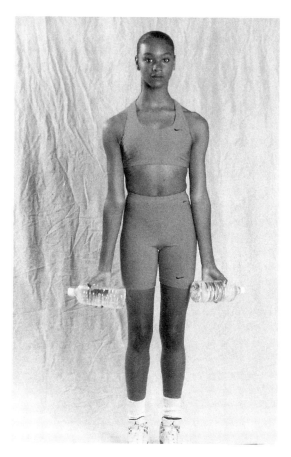

1. Begin by facing a step bench or the bottom of a flight of stairs. Hold a weight in each hand, with your arms hanging naturally by your side and your palms facing forward.

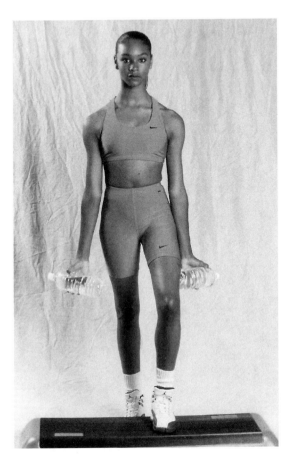

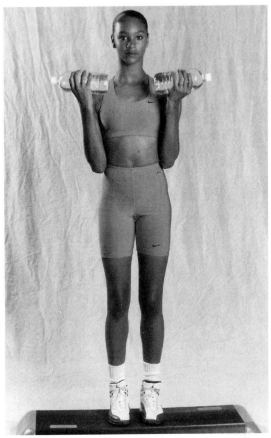

2. Step up with your left foot, and then step up with the right foot.

3. Curl both arms and bring the weights to shoulder level, keeping your wrists straight and your elbows at your side. Step down with your left foot first, followed by your right foot, then lower the weights to the starting position. Repeat the move starting with your right foot.

Side Lunge and Overhead Press (works the thighs, buttocks, shoulders and arms)

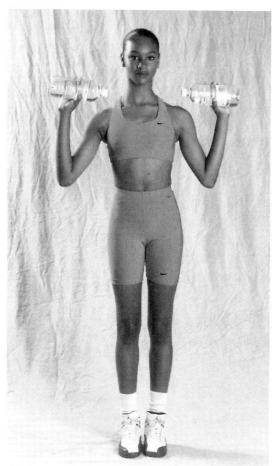

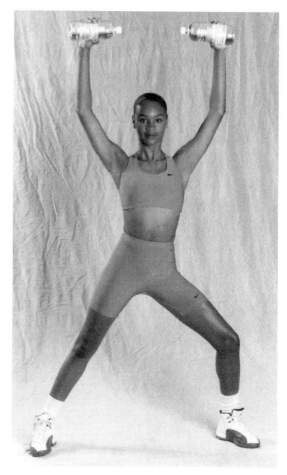

1. Stand with your feet slightly apart, holding weights in each hand, at shoulder level. Your palms should be facing forward.

2. Step into a side lunge position, leading with your left foot. Your left leg should be bent, with your knee over your heel and your right leg straight. As you lunge, press both arms overhead. Remember to keep your head up, your chest lifted, your shoulders pressed down, and your abdominals contracted. It's important not to arch your back during this exercise to prevent straining your muscles. Now step back to the starting position by pushing off with the heel of your left foot and lowering your arms. Repeat on the other side.

Seated Bent Over Row and Tricep Kickback (works the upper back, and back of the upper arm)

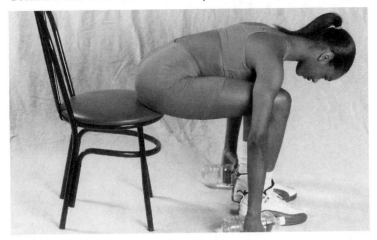

1. Start by sitting on the edge of a chair, feet flat on the floor hip width apart. Bend at the waist, and rest your chest on your thighs. Your arms should be hanging down along the outside of your legs, with weights in your hands and your palms facing inward.

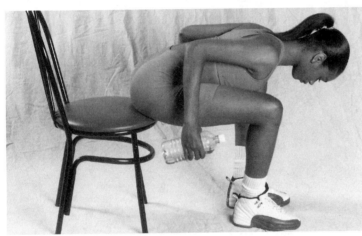

2. Squeezing your shoulder blades together (in order to have a more stable position to lift from), raise the weights straight up, leading with your elbows, keeping them close to your body.

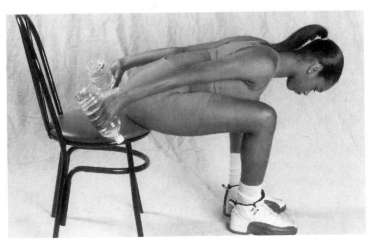

3. When the weights reach the sides of your thighs, extend your arms backward, leading with your hands. There should be no movement at the shoulders, only at the elbows (concentrate on keeping your upper arms motionless and parallel to the floor). After a pause, bend your arms in to return to the starting position.

Push-Up and Leg Curl (works the chest and arms, and back of the thigh)

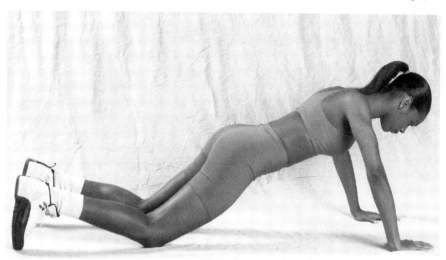

1. Start in a modified push-up position with your hands slightly wider than shoulder width, your head in alignment with the rest of your body, and your abs held in. Bend your elbows and lower your chest toward the floor.

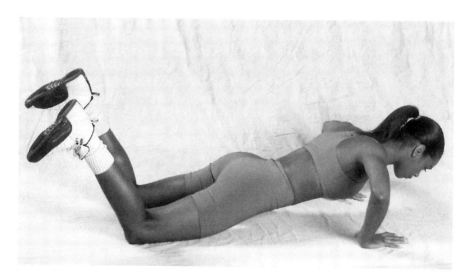

2. As you lower your body, slowly curl your legs by bending at the knees and bring your heels toward your buttocks. (If you wish, you can add resistance by using ankle weights to perform the leg curl.) Then straighten your arms, and lower your legs to return to the starting position. (Option: If you can't do a prone push-up, do a standing wall push-up, followed by a leg curl.)

Double Crunch (works the abdominals)

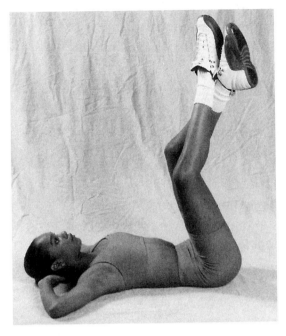 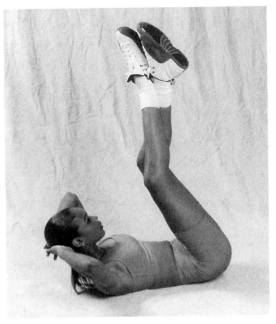

1. Lie on your back with your legs up, ankles crossed, and your knees bent over your hips. Place your hands behind your head so your fingers touch but don't interlock. Contract your abdominals, exhale, and bring your hips toward your rib cage while lifting your buttocks off the floor.

2. As you perform this movement (called a reverse curl), curl your upper body forward, and raise your shoulder blades off the floor. Exhale during the lifting stage. Avoid swinging your legs and pulling the back of your neck during the exercise. Return to the starting position by lowering both portions of your body at the same time to complete one rep.

Each of these exercises involves two separate exercises. As you do them, it's important to concentrate on your form. Start off by doing one set of eight to twelve repetitions, two to three times a week, with lighter weights. As you progress, you can work up to two to three sets, using heavier weights, three times a week.

Work It Out at Work

Now that you know how to get busy at home, I'm going to show you how you can get physical at the office. Doing these exercises (both strengthening and flexibility) will help relieve that chronic pain in your neck, and help stave off that mid-afternoon energy slump. (And if you didn't have time to fit in some strength training moves before you left the house, you can sneak them in from 9 to 5!) Each exercise should be repeated eight to twelve times.

Desk Push-Up (works the chest, front of shoulders and triceps)

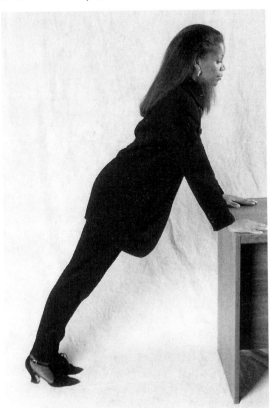 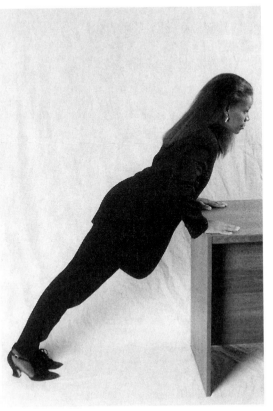

1. Lean forward and place your hands on top of your desk with your feet hip width apart. Your arms should be slightly beyond shoulder width. Your body should form a straight line from head to toe. Keep your abs contracted and avoid arching your back.

2. Lower your body toward the desk, then straighten your arms to return to the starting position. (Optional: This exercise can also be performed against a wall, or on a photocopier.)

Desk Dip (works the triceps)

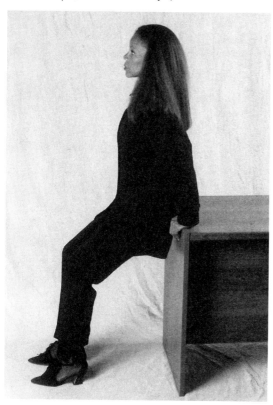 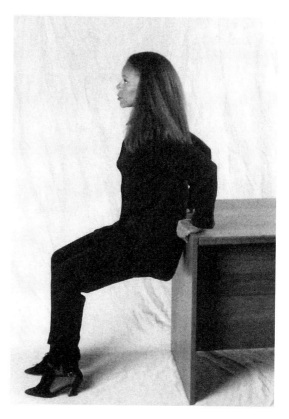

1. Stand facing away from a desk with your feet shoulder width apart, and your knees bent directly over your ankles. Place your hands on the edge of the desk behind you with your arms straight.

2. Lower your buttocks to knee level, then lift yourself back into the starting position by straightening your arms at the elbow.

Seated Bicep Curl (works the biceps)

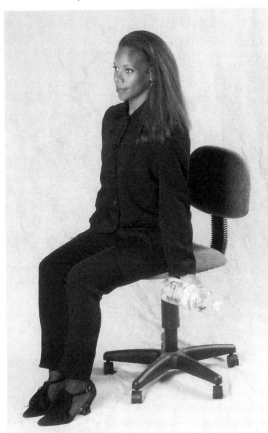
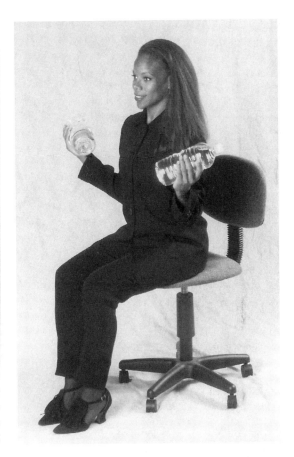

1. Sit on the edge of your chair with your abs in, your chest lifted and your shoulders relaxed. Your arms should be lowered at your side with weights (or water bottles) in your hands.

2. Lift the weights toward your shoulders by bending at the elbows. Keep your elbows close to your side, and keep your wrists straight. Lower to the starting position.

Shoulder Shrug (relieves muscle tension in the neck and shoulders)

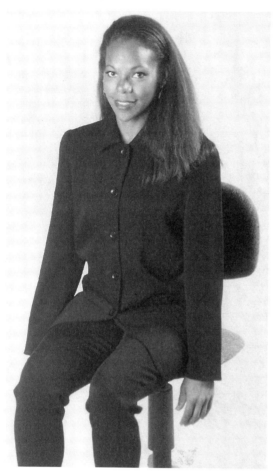 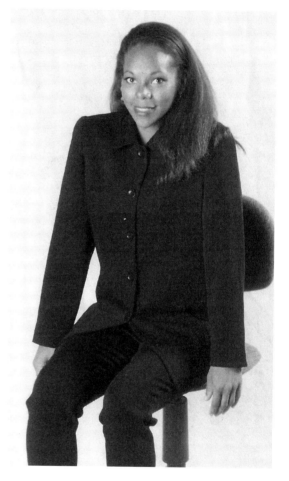

1. Sit erect in your chair, keeping your abdominals contracted, your chest lifted, and your shoulders down.

2. Lift your shoulders toward your ears, and pause at the top. Let the tension in your neck go by relaxing your shoulders down to the starting position. Repeat several times.

Back Stretch (helps relax back tension)

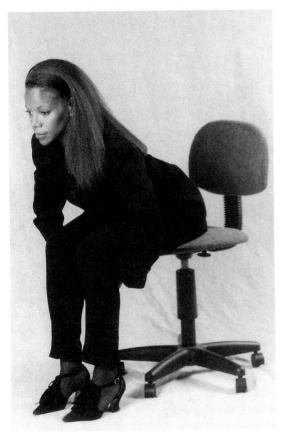 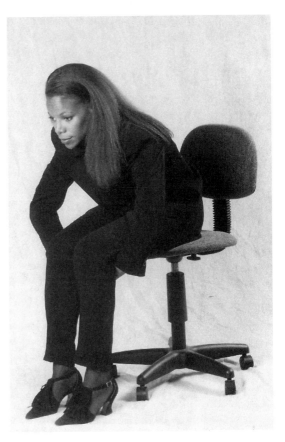

1. Sit in your chair and lower your chest toward your thighs. Keep your back straight, and place your hands under your thighs.

2. Contract your abs and round your back. Then return to starting position and repeat several times..

Neck Stretch (releases neck tension)

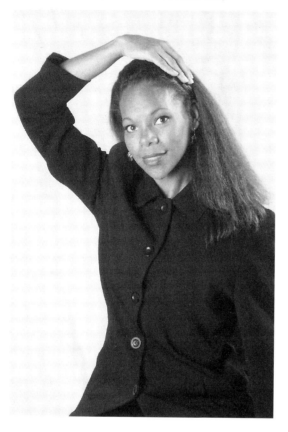 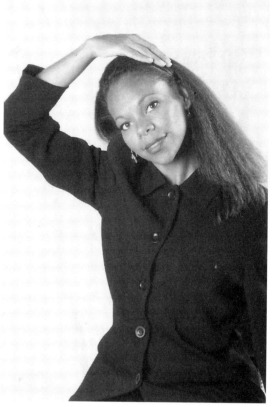

1. While sitting in your chair, bend your right arm overhead and place your right palm on the left side of your head.

2. Tilt your head and gently press down while reaching your left hand down toward the floor. Hold and repeat on the other side.

These aren't the only exercises you can do in the confines of your office. Small movements, such as circling your ankles, pointing and flexing your toes, performing a wrist bend (gently pulling back on your wrist with your opposite hand), and slowly rolling your head are great for relieving physical stress. In addition, you can even use funny faces to release facial tension or just grab a stress ball and squeeze, baby, squeeze. The idea is to let loose and destress. Of course, a more structured exercise program is the real key to remaining stress free and physically fit on a long-term basis, but we'll get to that in the coming chapters.

Cool It with Miss D

Don't forget to cool down after you work out. It's as essential as the warm-up component of your workout. After exercise (especially aerobics) your body is still in a revved-up mode. Your heart rate, blood pressure, and breathing are all higher than usual. The job of the cool down is to get the body to relax, gradually bringing the system back to normal. You want to do a low-intensity full-body movement—like walking at a moderate pace or gently marching in place—until your breathing returns to normal.

Now is also the perfect time to increase your flexibility. Because your muscles are nice and warm from working out, you'll be able to stretch them further—and hold the stretches longer—than you were able to do in the warm-up period. Doing light stretching before beginning any type of exercise is a good idea (after the brief warm-up, of course), but it's especially useful at the end of a workout. It helps prevent what's known as Delayed Onset Muscle Soreness, or D.O.M.S. What this means in English is that stretching today will keep you from aching tomorrow.

Performing a few light stretches helps bring the muscles back to their normal length, and it helps prevent that old stiff feeling that many people experience after a workout. The stretches are the same ones you did in the warm-up period (see photos on pages 26 to 28), but during the cool-down you hold them a bit longer—ten to thirty seconds—which will help keep your body supple, limber, and ready for action! (Personally, I like to stretch with my main squeeze, because it fees really good. I mean, it's nice to stretch each other out. I'm a big advocate of s-t-r-e-t-c-h-i-n-g it out, if you know what I mean.)

4

Stay Fit

Now that you've started to master the first stage of your fitness program, you're probably ready for a new challenge. You've already learned how to pick goals and how to set aside the time to achieve them, and you've begun to reap the benefits of an active lifestyle. Feels great, doesn't it? Finally. . . the moment you've all been waiting for (drumroll, please). . . it's time to learn the fundamentals of a structured, intermediate-level exercise program—the kind that will make you really fit and give you those killer abs and toned biceps that you've been dreaming of. All right, then, let me show you how to turn those dreams into reality!

Designing Your Intermediate GetFit Program

The intermediate stage of your fitness program (which lasts from fourteen to twenty-two weeks) will involve a different set of standards than those outlined in the previous chapter. Luckily, the American College of Sports Medicine (ACSM) has already done the work for us (bless their hearts!). When it comes to setting up a safe and effective program, the ACSM's Guidelines for Exercise Prescription are considered the gold standard in the fitness industry.

As in the beginner's program, the intermediate workout goals are divided into guidelines for aerobic exercise, weight training, and stretching sessions. For all of these components, the guidelines can be broken down into a principle that's known as F.I.T.T.: Frequency of the activity, Intensity of the activity, Time of the activity, and Type of activity. In other words: think F.I.T.T. to get fit. (Easy to remember, right?)

Types of Aerobic Exercise

The ACSM Guidelines for aerobic exercise are based on a total *time* of twenty to sixty minutes per session, for a *frequency* of three to five times a week, at an *intensity* of 60 to 80 percent of your maximum heart rate (in laymen's terms, that's the fastest your heart can beat), or 60 to 80 percent of what's called your "heart rate reserve" (which I'll explain in detail later in this chapter). What's great about the ACSM Guidelines is that they provide the basic parameters for our workout, but allow us to fill them in with whatever we want.

You have numerous choices in the *type* of aerobic exercise you can do during your workout. Exercises that consist of straight ahead movements—such as riding a stationary bike, using a cross-country ski machine, and running—are all good aerobic options. Another type of aerobic exercise consists of vertical movements: step aerobics, stair climbers, and incline treadmill walking. Finally, there's a newer form of aerobic exercise that involves lateral movements—such as slide training and in-line skating—which can be done alfresco on Rollerblades, or indoors on a skating machine or slide pad. Whatever form of cardiovascular exercise you choose to do, by this stage of the program, you should be working out aerobically for twenty to sixty minutes, three to five times a week.

By varying your program with these different types of aerobic exercises, you can train the muscles in your body from as many different angles as possible—which is why it's called cross-training. My favorite workouts include aerobics (of course!), power walking, in-line skating, dancing and hiking with friends. Cross-training is where it's at. Not only does it help keep you from getting bored and dropping out of your fitness routine, it also makes you better able to handle life's little twists and turns—literally. An executive stepping off the curb to hail a taxi, a housewife walking up a flight of stairs with some groceries, and an older adult slipping on a rug in her house all need protection from life's sudden surprises. Training your body in different directions can help get and keep you up and running. You don't want to find yourself in the position of the "I've fallen and I can't get up" lady, now do you? Then get up already, and let's get going . . .

FAT STATS

Calorie Chart for Various Activities

When it comes to burning calories, most of us want to get as much bang for our exercise buck as possible. This chart, based on figures provided by the American Council on Exercise (ACE), will give you an idea of how your favorite aerobic activities measure up on the fat-burning scale (which varies, depending on your weight):

Activity	Calories Burned in 30 Minutes			
	120 LB.	140 LB.	160 LB.	180 LB.
Aerobic Dance	222	258	294	333
Basketball	225	264	300	339
Bowling	36	42	48	57
Cycling (10 mph)	165	192	219	246
Dancing (social)	87	99	111	126
Gardening (vigorously)	150	177	201	225
Golf (pull/carry clubs)	138	162	186	210
Golf (power cart)	63	75	84	96
Hiking	135	156	180	201
Jogging (10-minute mile)	279	324	372	417
Mountain Biking	234	272	310	349
Rowing	193	224	256	287
Running (7-minute mile)	342	396	453	510
Sitting quietly	36	39	45	51

	120 LB.	140 LB.	160 LB.	180 LB.
Skating (ice and roller)	177	207	237	264
Skiing (cross-country)	225	264	300	339
Skiing (water and downhill)	171	198	228	255
Stair climbing	220	256	292	328
Swimming (crawl, moderate pace)	234	270	309	348
Tennis	180	207	237	267
Walking (12-minute mile)	195	228	261	291
Weight training (free weights or machines)	198	228	261	294

Exercise Intensity and Heart Rate

Now that you've chosen the types of aerobic activity you want to do, you need to keep track of the intensity of your workouts. The best way to do this is by using a heart rate monitor. You can find heart rate monitors at most sporting goods stores and specialty running shops for around $100. For those of you who think that a heart rate monitor is a needless expense, I'm here to tell you you're wrong. Trying to exercise without one is like trying to drive your car on the highway without a speedometer—you end up breaking the law. You'll end up either going too easy to get any benefits or—and this is actually more common—working out too hard for your own good.

Exercising too intensely can be harmful to your body. It uses more of your limited carbohydrate stores (the nutrients that your body needs to stay energized and work efficiently) and less of your unlimited fat supply. In other words, you wind up burning muscle mass, not fat! This is the reason why many people who begin structured exercise programs are not satisfied with the outcome of their efforts. They're working *really, really* hard, but they're not getting the results they want. Worst of all, they have *no* idea why. If you're trying to lose weight, you need to exercise at a lower intensity to burn fat.

After you've been exercising for a while, you can increase the frequency, intensity, and duration of your workout to keep your fitness routine challenging. In fact, some people swear by once-a-week interval training sessions, in which you alternate short bursts of intensive activity with longer periods of slower activity. Interval training helps increase your physical endurance and boost your metabolism. Research shows that a regular half-hour aerobic session boosts metabolism for about thirty minutes after exercising, while an interval session increases your metabolism for a whopping forty-eight hours afterward! But because it is harder on your body, fitness experts recommend that you utilize interval training no more than once a week.

For example, you might program a stationary bike for three minutes at a comfortable pace, then do one minute at a fast incline, then return to the slower pace for another three minutes, then speed it up for one minute, and so on, for a total of twenty to sixty minutes. The best way to experiment with interval training is by using the interval or hill program on a stationary bike, treadmill, or stair climber. Beginners should stick with the 3:1 ratio (three minutes slower activity combined with one minute at the faster pace). As you progress up the fitness ladder, you can switch to a 2:2 ratio, then move on to a 1:3 ratio (one minute slow activity, three minutes at a brisk pace) when you've become a more advanced exerciser.

In the beginning, though, it's not about working out hard—it's about working out *smart*. The smarter you work out, the less likely you are to injure yourself, and the more likely you are to exercise for longer periods of time and to stick with the program over the long haul. And when it comes to getting and staying fit, consistency is what it's all about. (It's the old "use it or lose it" principle.)

Taking Your Pulse

If you still don't want to invest in a heart rate monitor, all hope is not lost. There are two methods of taking your pulse the old-fashioned way: by your wrist, or by the carotid artery on your neck. Both ways have their advantages and disadvantages.

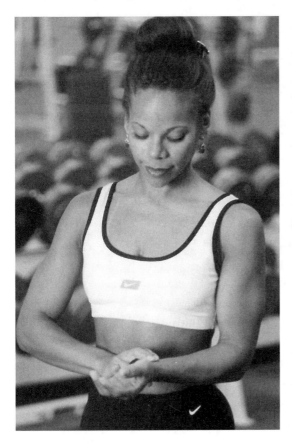

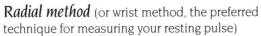

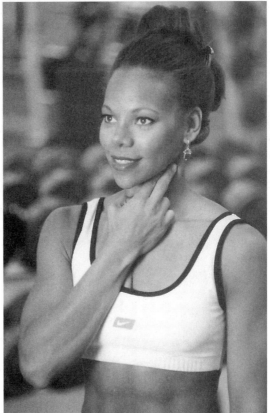

Radial method (or wrist method, the preferred technique for measuring your resting pulse)

Place the index and middle fingers of your right hand on the outside of your left forearm, near the point where it meets the base (palm) of your hand. Making sure that your fingers are in line with the bottom of your thumb, apply light pressure. Count the number of beats for a full minute. (It is important not to use your thumb, because it has a pulse of its own and can, therefore, produce an inaccurate reading.)

Carotid method (the preferred technique for measuring your exercise pulse rate)

Place the index and middle fingers of your right hand on the right side of your neck, adjacent to your larynx (voice box), just under your jaw. Using light pressure, count the number of beats for ten seconds. Multiply this number by six to get the total number of beats per minute.

The radial (wrist) method is more difficult to perform during exercise, but some people can show a lower heart rate when the pulse is taken at the carotid artery—especially if they apply too much pressure to the artery. Experiment with both methods to determine which method is easier for you.

Figuring Out Your Training Heart Rate

There are also two ways to determine your training heart rate. The most common method is to use a simple mathematical formula (220 minus your age for men, and 226 minus your age for women) to figure out your maximum heart rate, then multiply that number by 60% (the low end of the aerobic target zone) and again by 80% (the high end of the target zone). So, in the case of a forty-year-old woman, it would look like this (I've rounded off the numbers to keep things simple):

1. $226 - 40 = 186$
2. $186 \times 60\%$ (low end of aerobic target zone) $= 112$
3. $186 \times 80\%$ (high end of aerobic target zone) $= 149$

So a forty-year-old woman should aim to have her heart beat between 112 and 149 beats per minute during a workout. If her hearbeat dips below 112, she's not working hard enough, and if it goes above 149, she's exerting too much effort and should slow down. This formula, however, only gives you an *estimate* of how hard you should be working, since it doesn't take into account the individual's resting pulse rate—which can vary wildly from person to person.

Top fitness experts use another method, called the Karvonen Formula, to determine a client's exact target zone. This is the method that I recommend you use to figure out your training heart rate. Unlike the age-only method, the Karvonen Formula is more accurate because it figures in the individual's resting heart rate (the number of times your heart beats per minute when you're sitting still). Including your resting heart rate into the calculations allows you to individualize the equation, since it's a good indicator of what shape you're in at that time. A slim, moderately active thirty-year-old woman, for instance, will probably have a very different resting pulse rate than an over-weight, inactive woman of the same age. For a healthy woman who's not on any type of medication, the lower her resting heart rate, the better her fitness level. The opposite holds true as well. Why is this so?

Because your heart is a muscle. Just like any other muscle, it can become stronger through exercise and better at doing its job—pumping blood. Ideally, a heart should beat less and pump more blood at a lower rate. If you're out of shape, though, your heart will beat faster but pump less blood in the process.

If you want to figure out your *exact* training heart rate you have to subtract your resting pulse rate from your maximum heart rate, to get what is called your "heart rate reserve." (There is a little more figuring involved in the Karvonen Formula, but don't worry, I'll walk you through it step by step. And it's all simple math—*no calculus*—I promise!) Once you've figured out your maximum heart rate, determine your resting pulse rate by using the radial or carotid method to see how many times your heart beats in sixty seconds (you can also count the beats for ten seconds and multiply by six). So if our forty-year-old example had a resting pulse of, say, seventy beats per minute, her Karvonen equation would look like this (again, I've rounded off the numbers):

1. Find your maximum heart rate:
   $226 - 40 = 186$ (226 minus your age)
2. Find your heart rate reserve:
   $186 - 70 = 116$ (maximum heart rate − resting pulse rate)
3. Multiply your heart rate reserve by 60%, then add your resting pulse rate back in:
   $116 \times 60\% = 70$ (heart rate reserve × low end of aerobic training zone)
   $70 + 70 = 140$
   140 is the low end of your heart rate reserve training zone
4. Multiply your heart rate reserve by 80%, then add your resting pulse rate back in:
   $116 \times 80\% = 93$ (heart rate reserve x high end of aerobic training zone)
   $93 + 70 = 163$
   163 is the high end of your heart rate reserve training zone

As you can see, the Karvonen method offers slightly different results than the age-only formula (a target range of 112 to 149 versus a target range of 140 to 163), which means our fictitious forty-year-old wouldn't be working out as hard as she should be if she used the age-only formula to determine her training zone.

As I've already mentioned, according to the ACSM Guidelines, technically you can use between 60 to 80 percent of your heart rate reserve (or 60 percent to 80 percent of your maximum heart rate) during your exercise program. My advice? Those of you who are just starting out should stay in the 60 to 70 percent range, with only serious exercisers going over 80 percent. If you stick to these guidelines, you'll see better results in the way of fat loss and will be less prone to injury and burnout.

Aerobics Made Easy

When doing any type of cardiovascular exercise, you want to slowly increase the duration of your workouts every couple of weeks until you can do at least twenty minutes nonstop. To keep from overdoing it, remember to use the 10 Percent Rule. Don't ever increase the total time or total miles that you work out by over 10 percent of the previous week's total. Continue to use the 10 Percent Rule to build up the time of your workouts as you progress in your program. It will help prevent both overexertion and dropout.

In addition to the 10 Percent Rule, it helps to include a day of rest in between your aerobic workouts. When you're starting out, it will help keep you going. Your schedule might look something like this:

MONDAY	TUESDAY	WEDNESDAY	THURSDAY	FRIDAY
Walk	Rest	Bike	Rest	Walk

Pump, Pump, Pump It Up!

Following the same F.I.T.T. equation for weight training, the ACSM recommends that you include at least two sessions of weight training per week. (I recommend that you weight train at least three to four times a week if you really want to see results.) During those sessions, do one set of eight to ten different exercises, for eight to twelve repetitions each. In a month or two, when doing one set becomes too easy, you can up it to two—and eventually three—sets of each exercise (at eight to twelve reps each).

Here you also have a choice of the type of resistive training equipment that you can use: free weights, weight machines, rubber tubing, and weighted bars are all possibilities. Each piece of equipment has its own advantages and disadvantages. For example, free weights help build better body awareness, in the form of balance and coordination. On the other hand, weight machines are easy to use, force you to use proper form, and can be combined in a circuit-training program to give you maximum benefits in a shorter period of time. Rubber tubing is another option that's great to use at home or when you're traveling because it's lightweight and easy to store.

Designing a Balanced Program

When designing a weight training program, you want to make sure that you balance the strength between all the muscle groups in your body. Many people make the mistake of concentrating only on the areas that they want to improve. For example, some women think that if they train their thighs, their legs will automatically become slim and trim. The real truth is that you can't spot reduce. The only way to get rid of extra weight on your body is through a sound program of exercise and healthy eating. I recommend using a combination of fat-burning aerobic exercise along with some metabolism-boosting muscle-sculpting weight training.

There's another problem that you'll run into if you only train your "trouble" spots—injury. Any time you work one muscle group (such as the bicep in the front of the arm) you *must* work the opposite muscle group (in this case, the tricep in the back of the arm). By designing a program that promotes good overall balance, not only will your body function better, you will also be less apt to hurt yourself.

Weight Training Systems

There are several different systems or routines that can you can use to increase muscular strength and endurance. The basic concept to understand is this: heavier weights and fewer repetitions will develop your strength (and increase the size of your muscle), while lighter weights and more repetitions will train your muscle endurance (and build muscle tone without bulk). Some of the more popular strength-training systems include:

Multiple sets. This is the most commonly used form of training. It consists of performing numerous sets (two or more) for as many as ten to twelve repetitions.

Circuit training. Consists of a series of ten to fourteen exercises done one after another, with minimal rest (about thirty seconds) between exercises. This type of routine improves muscle endurance, using light weights and a greater number of repetitions (ten to fifteen).

Single sets. Used frequently in circuit training, where you complete only one set of each exercise. Although it doesn't appear to produce the same benefits as the multiple set method in the long run, it's great for people who are pressed for time.

Split routine. This type of program is used a lot by body-builders. Multiple sets and multiple exercises for each individual body part are performed in an effort to bulk up (hypertrophy). Most serious weight trainers break up or "split" their routine by doing exercises for the upper body on Mondays and Thursdays, and movements for the lower body on Tuesdays and Fridays. Such a schedule is very time-consuming, and it is not recommended for the average person.

Super sets. Involves combining several exercises together, with little rest in between, with eight to ten repetitions on each movement. You can perform a super set by using two exercises that work the same body part (such as standing curls and seated preacher curls for the biceps), or by choosing exercises that work opposing muscle groups (like leg extensions for your quadriceps and leg curls for your hamstrings).

Pyramiding. Uses ascending (light to heavy), or descending (heavy to light) progressions during the exercise you are performing. For example, you might start off with sixty pounds on the bench and go to seventy, and then eighty. Or you might reverse the process and move down from eighty to seventy to sixty. (The heavy-to-light method shows the best gains in strength.)

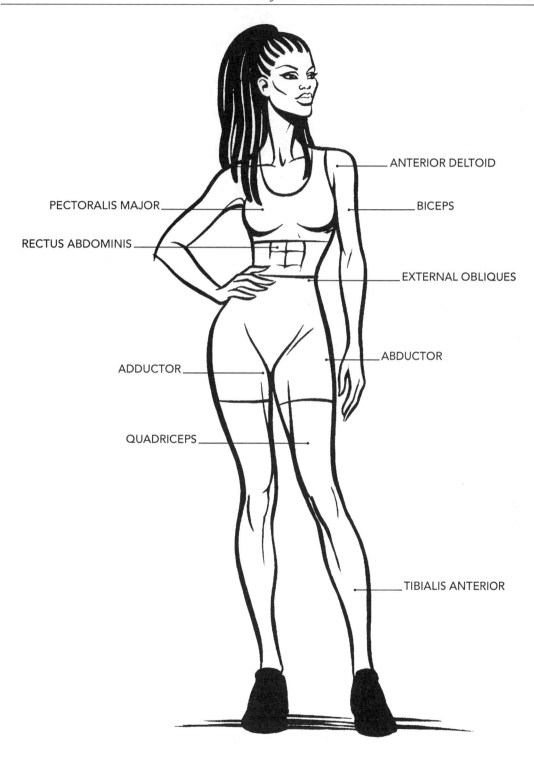

ANTERIOR DELTOID

PECTORALIS MAJOR

BICEPS

RECTUS ABDOMINIS

EXTERNAL OBLIQUES

ADDUCTOR

ABDUCTOR

QUADRICEPS

TIBIALIS ANTERIOR

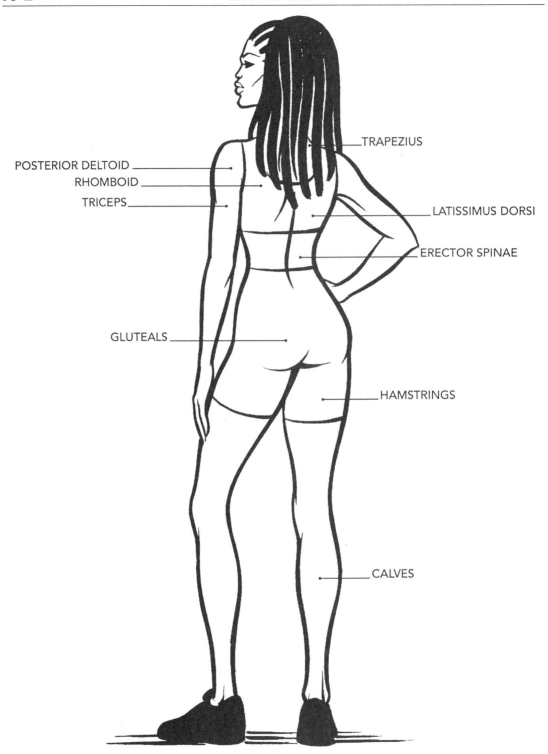

POSTERIOR DELTOID

RHOMBOID

TRICEPS

TRAPEZIUS

LATISSIMUS DORSI

ERECTOR SPINAE

GLUTEALS

HAMSTRINGS

CALVES

Muscle Groups and Weight Training Exercises

Miss Donna is always working to make things easier for you. To help match up the muscles you want to work with the proper exercise, I've developed this easy-to-read chart. In an effort to get maximum benefits, I have picked exercises that work the same muscle group from different angles (think of it as cross-training for your muscles). I'll explain how to do each exercise a little later on (although you'll want to consult your friendly training staff when using any machines at the gym).

Muscle Group	Barbells	Machines
Buttocks	Squat Lunge	Leg Press Hack Squat Glute/Ham Developer
Quadriceps (front of thigh)	Squat Lunge	Leg Extension Hack Squat Leg Press
Hamstring (back of thigh)	Squat Lunge	Leg Curl Hack Squat Leg Press
Calves	Calf Raise	Standing Calf Raise Seated Calf Raise
Inner Thigh	Side Lunge	Multi-Hip Adductor Machine Low Cable Adduction
Outer Thigh	Side Lunge	Multi-Hip Abductor Machine Low Cable Abduction
Pectoralis major (chest)	Bench Press Dumbbell flys Incline Press	Vertical Chest Press "Pec Deck" Nautilus Decline Press
Latissimus Dorsi (back)	Bent Over Row Bent Arm Pullover	"Lat" Pulldown Pullover Pull-up Station

Muscle Group	Barbells	Machines
Deltoids (shoulders)	Seated Press Front Raise Side Raise Bent Over Rear Raise	Seated Overhead Press Lateral Raise
Biceps (front of arm)	Standing Curl Preacher Curl Incline Dumbbell Curl	Bicep Curl
Tricep (back of arm)	Lying Tricep Extension "French Curl" Tricep "Kickbacks"	Tricep Pushdown Tricep Extension Dip Station

Muscle Imbalances

As I've previously stated, it's important to keep the body in balance by equally working all of the major muscles groups during your strength training program. (You don't want to be lopsided, now do you?!) Here are some of the more common imbalances that can occur during a weight lifting program. The important thing is to work out opposing muscle groups:

Stronger and More Inflexible Muscles	Weaker Muscles
Gastrocnemius (calf)	Tibialis Anterior (shin)
Quadriceps (front of thigh)	Hamstrings (back of thigh)
Abductors (outside of thigh)	Adductors (inside of thigh)
Erector Spinae (low back)	Abdominals (stomach)
Pectorals (chest)	Trapezius(upper back)
Biceps (front of arm)	Triceps (back of arm)

Real Women DO *Pump* Iron!

A problem I often face when working with women who weight train is getting them to understand that they will *not* become female Sylvester Stallones. It's just not possible to become overly muscle-bound unless you spend every waking hour in the gym pumping iron. Women don't have testosterone, so there's no way we can get as big as men.

I lift weights as part of my own personal fitness program, and I feel stronger and more confident. In addition to making you look great, weight training is a great way to help prevent osteoporosis and to generally improve posture through increased muscle control. (Your muscles help support important structures in your body such as your spine. If they're weak, slouching can result. And don't you want to stand tall?) Weight training also helps raise your metabolism, since muscle is more metabolically active than fat. This is good news for people who are trying to lose weight as a part of their fitness goal. With the additional lean body weight added in muscle, you'll walk around during the day with a higher metabolism and burn more calories while doing the same daily activities. It sounds too good too be true, but it's a fact, Jack!

Sculpting Your Body

I'm often asked what people can do about a pear-shaped body, where the lower body is bigger than the upper body. (It's what our grandmothers used to call "childbearing hips." Great for birthin' babies, not so great if you want to wear slim cut pants.) This problem usually results from a combination of a wide bone structure in the hips, compounded by extra body weight (fat) in the buttocks and thighs.

Weight training can be used to artistically shape the body into what you want it to be. Just as Michelangelo could look at a block of stone and see the sculpture he wanted to create, so can you visualize the body you want within your mind. Strength training can help you achieve the body you want—within limits. While you can reshape your body—sometimes dramatically—you still have to work with what Mother Nature gave you.

To help women who are pear-shaped (the most common female body type), I devise ways for them to add more muscle to their upper bodies. I start by assigning exercises for their shoulders, particularly for the middle portion, which tends to give added width to the body. This musculature takes away the visual emphasis from the hips, making the body shape look more symmetrical. Adding more muscle in the back area also creates a nice taper from the shoulders to the waist. Again, this helps create a more symmetrical shape, removing the visual impact of wide hips.

As I've already mentioned, if you follow a well-designed program, you will *not* get big and bulky. Instead, you'll end up with a lean, toned body. Just look at the physiques of people like Angela Bassett and Goldie Hawn (who, at age fifty-two, is definitely hittin' and holdin'). Many celebrities weight train, and they look amazing. Strong *is* sexy. Women who lift weights love to wear off-the-shoulder dresses, sleeveless shirts, and bathing suits. They're proud of their well-toned bodies and want to show them off. Hey, girlfriends, you *should* be proud of what you got!

I've developed a weight training routine for you to use during this stage of your fitness program. It's a free weight program consisting of eleven exercises that will work all of your major muscles and help you tone up and trim down. I'm telling you, this routine will have you looking mighty fine in no time.

The first thing you need to know about doing your program is how fast to lift the weight. Usually, I see people who lift too fast, which can increase the chance of injury. It's also not as effective as using slow, controlled movements. Don't just go through the motions—really involve yourself in the process. If you let the weight drop back down quickly, you're only working half of the movement, skipping what we fitness pros call the "lengthening" phase. Count to two while raising a weight during the "shortening" phase, and then lower it for a four count during the lengthening phase.

It's actually possible to overcome the weight of a barbell, or dumbbell, by using too much momentum. (In simple terms, you're cheating by *throwing* the weight up instead of lifting it in a slow, controlled manner.) Once you get a weight moving in the beginning of the exercise, it doesn't take much effort to keep it going. It's sort of like pushing a big boulder down a hill: it may take some effort to get it moving, but once momentum takes over, it doesn't require much work to keep it rolling. If you throw the weight around forcefully, your muscle isn't working to maximum capacity and you're not going to get the same amount of tone and definition that you'd get by using slow, deliberate movements.

Another important thing is to *know* how to breathe. I know you know how to breathe—you're still reading this, right? You haven't keeled over because you forgot how to draw breath, have you? But weight lifting demands a special kind of breathing. A lot of people hold their breath while they're lifting because they're concentrating so hard. But this can dramatically increase the pressure in your chest, causing what is known as the "Valsalva maneuver." When this happens, the blood pressure rises to dangerous levels. *This is not a good thing.*

You can achieve the best (and safest) results by waiting to exhale until you get to the hardest part of the lift, which is known as the "sticking point." At that time, your muscles may start to feel like they're quivering because they're working at their max. If you breathe out at this point, you can help relax your muscles, moving right through the sticking point. (This doesn't mean you should hold your breath during the exercise but that you should exhale during the most difficult point of the lift and inhale while you relax.)

Other basic tips to follow during your strength training program include the use of a weight belt. Wearing a weight belt helps support your back (especially when you're performing unsupported exercises using free weights). You also might want to buy a pair of lifting gloves. The last thing you want to do is chew up your hands with cold, hard steel.

Free Weights

The basic routine consists of two sets of eight to twelve repetitions, with a rest of one and a half to two minutes between sets, and three minutes between each exercise. When you start to feel stronger, add another set to each exercise until you have three total sets for every movement. To achieve optimum results, vary the exercises you do for each body part every other workout. For example, you can do squats for your legs one day and lunges the next. This will help build and balance the different muscle groups. You should aim to do this routine a minimum of two times a week.

The eleven basic exercises I've included have been designed to work your legs, chest, back, shoulders, biceps, triceps, and abdominals (in that order). In strength training it's important to always work from the larger muscle groups to the smaller ones. Working smaller muscles (such as the biceps) before you train a larger muscle group (like the "lats" in your back) makes it more difficult for you to perform the movement. (This is because the biceps are already fatigued before you even look to them to help work your back.)

It should take about forty-five minutes to do the free weight exercises I've chosen for your routine. (If you work out at a gym, ask a trainer to walk you through this routine the first time you do it, to make sure your form is correct.)

Squats (strengthens gluteus maximus, hamstrings, and quadriceps)

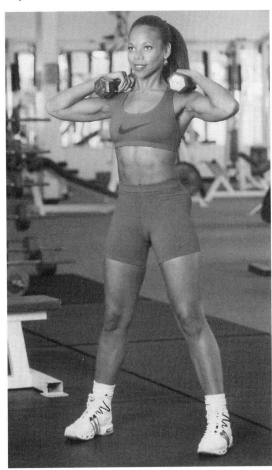 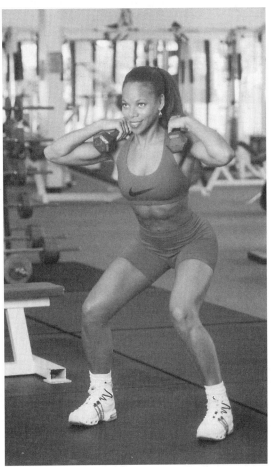

1. Stand with your feet parallel and slightly beyond shoulder-width apart, toes pointed forward. Hold the dumbbells at shoulder level, elbows bent and palms facing inward. Contract your abdominals and press your tailbone toward the floor.

2. Keeping your back straight, bend your knees and lower your buttocks as if you're going to sit down in a chair, keeping your knees over your heels. Press your heels firmly into the floor and straighten your legs to starting position without locking your knees.

Lunges (strengthens buttocks, quadriceps, hamstrings, and calves)

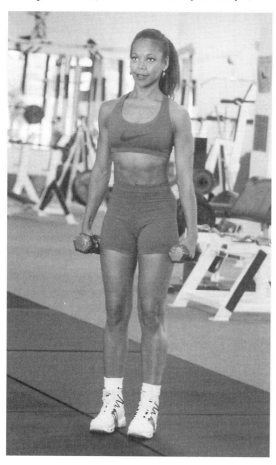 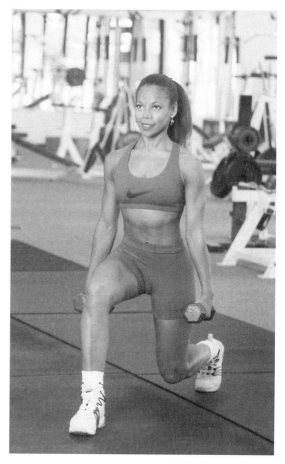

1. Hold a dumbbell in each hand and stand with your legs hip-width apart, arms at your sides, palms facing in.

2. Lunge forward with your right leg until your thigh is parallel with the floor and your knee is over your ankle. Your left leg should be trailing behind you, with your knee bent. Push off with your right foot to return to the starting position. Perform all reps, then switch legs.

Seated Calf Raises (strengthens calf muscles)

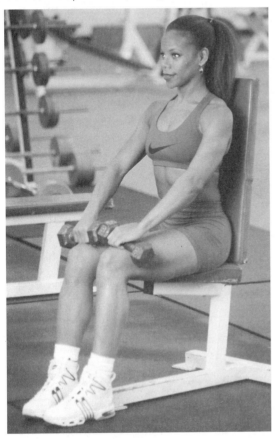 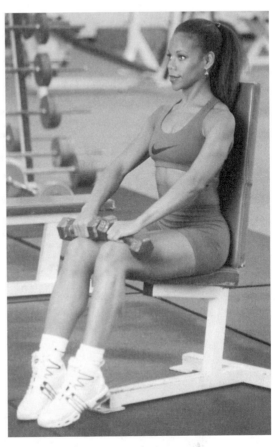

1. Sit on a flat bench or chair so that your lower legs form a 90-degree angle.

2. Hold the dumbbells on top of your thighs close to your knees, and raise your heels off the floor. Pause in the raised position, then lower your heels back to the floor.

Bench Press (strengthens pectorals, anterior deltoids, and triceps)

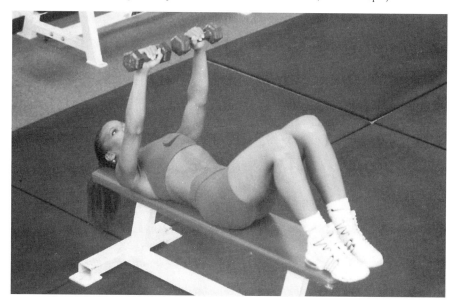

1. Lie on your back on a bench, with your knees bent and your feet flat on the bench. Holding a dumbbell in each hand, extend your arms straight above your chest with palms facing forward.

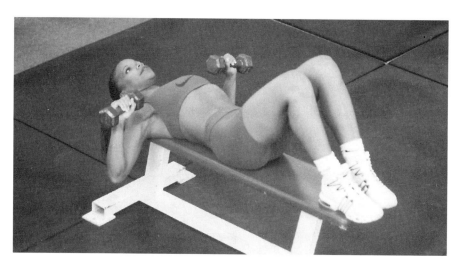

2. Keeping your abdominals tight and your lower back in contact with the bench, bend your elbows out and down until your upper arms are in line with your shoulders and the weights are parallel with the side of your chest. Straighten your arms to the starting position.

Bentover Row (strengthens latissimus dorsi, rhomboids, trapezius, and posterior deltoids)

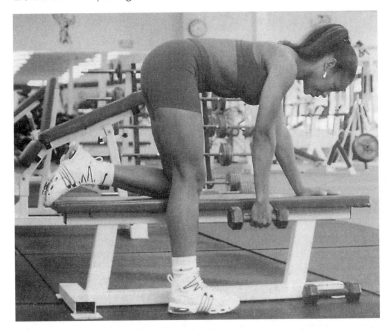

1. Hold a dumbbell in your right hand, and rest the lower part of your left leg flat against a bench. Keeping your right knee slightly bent, bend forward at the waist so that your back is parallel with the floor and the bench. Your left hand should be flat on the bench for support, your right arm should extend down toward the floor, palm facing in.

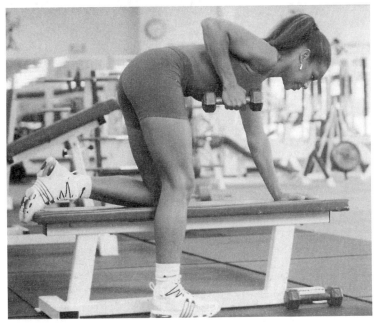

2. Squeeze your shoulder blades together and lift until the dumbbell is in line with the side of your chest. Hold for a count of two, then slowly straighten your right arm back to the starting position (but don't lock your elbow). Do all reps, then switch sides (right leg on bench, weight in left hand) and repeat.

Overhead Press (strengthens deltoids and triceps)

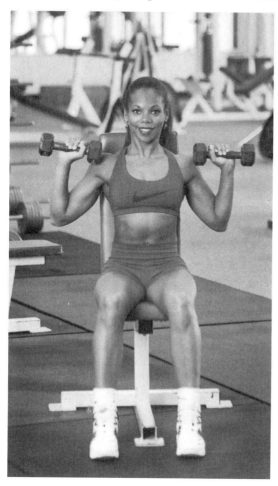 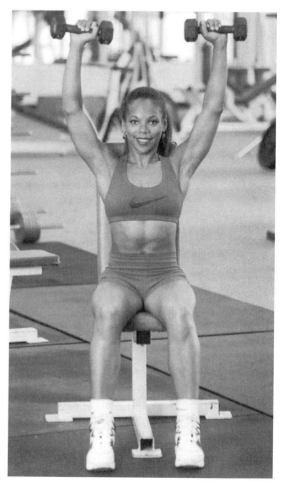

1. Sit with your back pressed flat against a bench or chair and your feet firmly on the floor, holding dumbbells at shoulder level, palms facing out.

2. Press the weights up, keeping your elbows slightly bent (the dumbbells should be slightly in front of—not directly over—your head). Lower the weights back down to shoulder level.

Seated One-Arm Dumbbell Curl (strengthens biceps)

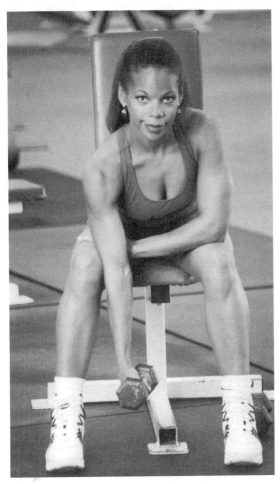 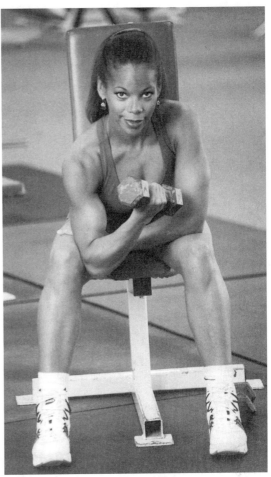

1. Sit on a flat bench or chair with your heels shoulder-width apart and your toes pointing forward. Hold a dumbbell in your right hand, and place your right elbow against your right knee.

2. Curl the dumbbell toward your shoulder, pause at the top, then return to starting position. Do all reps before switching sides.

Tricep Kickback (strengthens triceps)

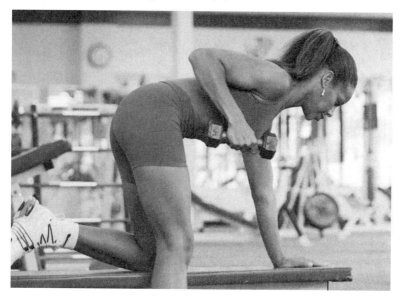

1. Hold a weight in your right hand, and rest the lower part of your left leg flat against a bench. Keeping your right knee slightly bent, lean over from the waist so that your back is parallel with the floor and the bench. Your left hand should be flat on the bench for support, and the upper part of your right arm should be parallel to the floor, with the weight next to your chest.

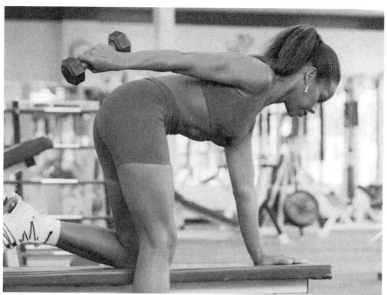

2. Keeping your upper arm close to your body, extend the weight back until your entire arm is straight and parallel with the floor. You should only move the lower part of your arm (from the elbow down) during this exercise; your upper arm should remain motionless. Bend your elbow to bring the weight back in toward your chest. Do all reps, then switch sides and repeat on the other arm.

Back Extension (strengthens erector spinae muscles)

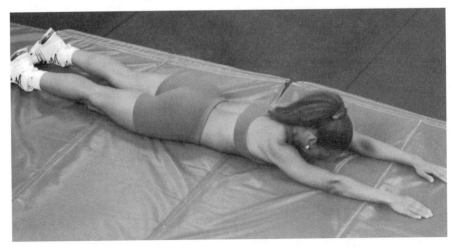

1. Lie facedown on the floor with a towel folded under your hips. Keep your abdominals contracted and place your arms straight overhead with your hands resting on the floor.

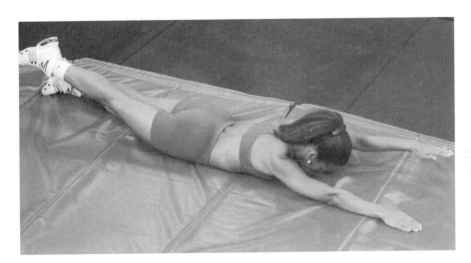

2. Slowly raise your left arm and right leg off of the floor. Hold for a few seconds, then lower to starting position. Do all reps, then repeat on other side.

Abdominal Crunch (works the rectus abdominus)

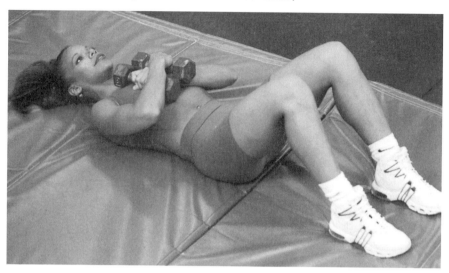

1. This exercise can be done with or without weights. Lie on your back, knees bent and feet flat on the floor. If you want to use weights, hold a dumbbell in each hand with your arms crossed over your chest.

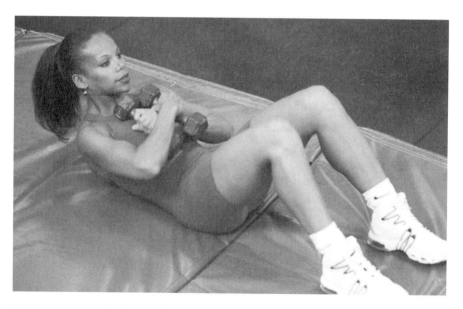

2. Contract your abdominals and curl your head, neck and shoulders up and forward as you exhale. Your shoulder blades should come up off the floor, but your lower back should stay in contact with it. Pause at the top, then lower your body to the starting position.

Side Crunch (works external obliques)

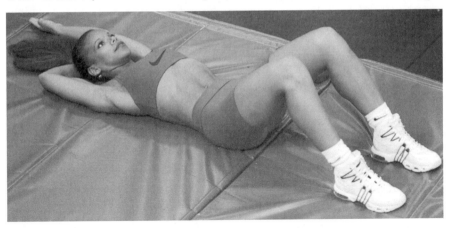

1. Lie on your back with your knees bent and your feet flat on the floor. Extend your left arm overhead, bend your right arm and place your right hand under your left upper arm.

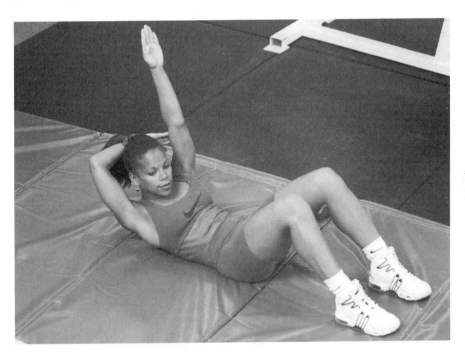

2. As you contract your abdominals, exhale and lift and rotate your upper body so that your left shoulder points toward your right knee. Pause for a moment, then lower your body to the starting position. Do all reps, then repeat on the other side. (Optional: Place both hands behind your head or crossed in front of your chest to make the movement less challenging.)

Setting Up Your Total Fitness Program

There are two different ways to add cardiovascular exercise to your strength training program. The first way involves killing two birds with one stone: include it on the same day that you perform your strength training workout. It really doesn't matter which one you do first. If you want to concentrate on getting in a good lift, do that first (just make sure to warm up beforehand by starting out with lighter weights or by doing some light cardio, like walking or riding the stationary bike for five minutes). If you want to have a great cardio workout, then start with that component. I like to alternate my activities every other workout anyway, including changing the type of aerobic exercise I do. I may jog one day, ride the stationary bike the next, and box the day after that. So my routine looks something like this:

Monday	Wednesday	Friday
Weights	Bike	Weights
Jog	Weights	Boxing

Once you've stuck to this schedule for several months, you might consider adding more days to your training routine. Alternate your cardiovascular exercise with your strength training work as follows (and make sure you avoid weight training the same muscle groups two days in a row, as muscles need at least twenty-four hours of rest between workouts in order to repair themselves):

	Monday	Tuesday	Wednesday	Thursday	Friday
Week One:	Weights	Bike	Weights	Jog	Weights
Week Two:	Climber	Weights	Walk	Weights	Swim

Just make sure that you take at least one day off a week. (Hey, even the Big Guy rested on the seventh day!)

Stretch It Out!

When it comes to increasing your flexibility, there are several different methods that get the job done. The most common form of stretching is the static stretch. Stretches of this type require that you hold a specific position for a set period of time, usually ten to thirty seconds, to help provide a good controlled stretch.

Another type of stretching is called PNF, or proprioceptive neuromuscular facilitation (don't worry about how to pronounce it—just know what it is). It involves a technique known as "contract and relax," which has been proven more effective than conventional stretching methods. If you wanted to stretch your hamstrings, for example, you would isometrically contract (or squeeze) the muscle for about ten seconds, then perform a gentle stretch to help cause a relaxation reflex. This can be accomplished by pressing against a towel wrapped around your leg, or by pressing against a partner's shoulder. Finally, ballistic stretching uses rhythmical bouncing movements of the body to create momentum to stretch the muscle. It is a high-risk form of stretching, but it is appropriate for certain sports. It develops dynamic flexibility for explosive activities such as martial arts.

Both the PNF and ballistic methods are more advanced forms of stretching that require proper technique and adequate practice to be performed correctly. Static stretching, on the other hand, requires no assistance, takes little time to learn, and has a higher safety factor for those just starting out on a structured exercise program. (In other words, static stretching is your *friend*.)

In accordance with the ACSM guidelines, you should try to stretch at least three times a week. Hold each stretch between ten and thirty seconds to a point of mild discomfort, and repeat each stretch three to five times. (Keep in mind that "mild discomfort" is not the same as "screaming pain." You'll probably feel some muscle tightness during the beginning of a stretch, but if it *really* hurts, don't do it.)

Additionally, a good stretching program should include enough exercises to stretch all of the major muscle groups in the body while taking about ten to fifteen minutes to perform. Never bounce while you stretch, and always focus in on your breathing and remember to exhale while you are performing the stretching movement. Proper breathing helps relax the muscle farther so you get a better stretch.

Although I know plenty of folks who don't stretch after a workout, I think this is a big mistake. I love finishing up my workout by stretching out the muscles that just worked so hard for me. In fact, sometimes during a particularly difficult workout (yes, even I have difficult workouts—now and then), I find myself thinking of my finishing stretches as a reward for a job well done! It feels *sooo* good. Try it—you can thank me later.

Let's S-T-R-E-T-C-H!

These stretches will help prevent muscle injuries and will increase your overall flexibility. Hold each stretch for ten to thirty seconds. Take it nice and easy—and don't bounce!

Lower Back Stretch

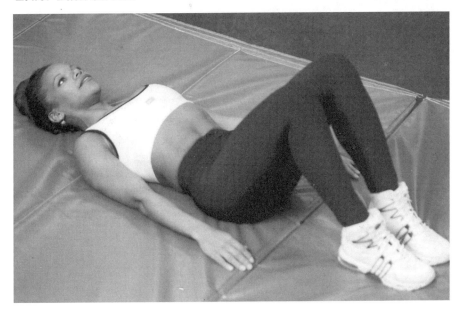

1. Lie on your back with your knees bent and your feet flat on the floor.

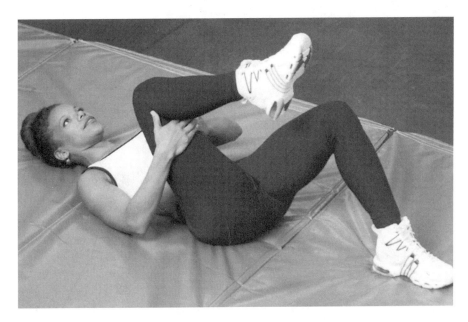

2. Bend your right leg, place both hands behind your thigh, and pull it toward your chest. Keep your back flat on the floor, concentrating the stretch on the back of your thigh, and hip. Repeat on the opposite leg.

Hamstring Stretch

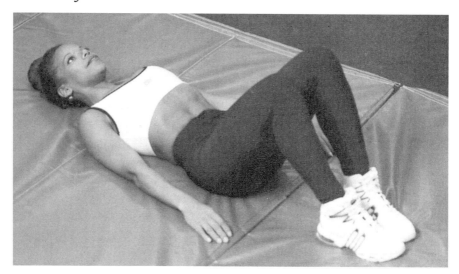

1. Lie on your back with your knees bent and your feet flat on the floor.

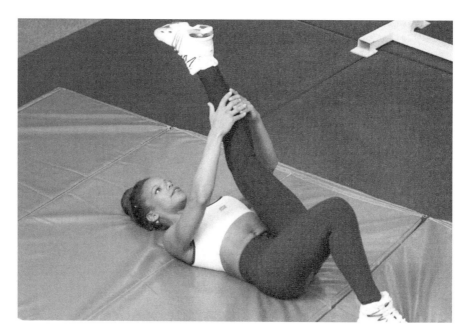

2. Bend your right leg, extend it straight in the air (keeping your knee slightly bent). Wrap your hands behind your calf, and pull it towards your chest. Keep your leg straight and your back in contact with the floor. Hold and repeat on the other leg.

Outer Hip Stretch

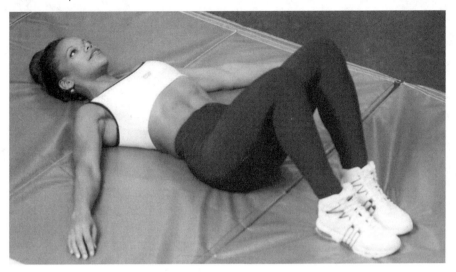

1. Lie on your back with your knees bent and your feet flat on the floor.

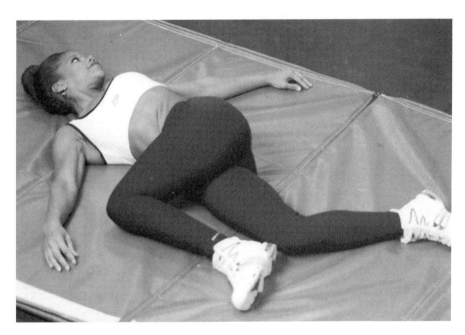

2. Bend your left knee and raise it toward your torso while extending your right leg out on the mat. Pull your left knee down and across your body. Keep your head and shoulders flat on the floor so that you feel the stretch across your outer hip and thigh. Relax and repeat on the right side.

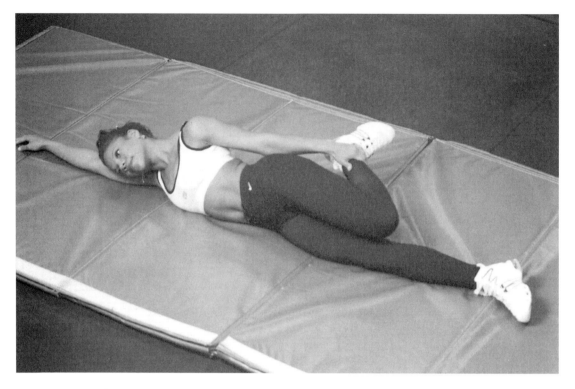

Quadriceps Stretch

1. Lie on your right side with your legs extended out and your right arm extended overhead. Bend your left leg back and grasp the top of your foot with your left hand. Gently pull your leg up toward your buttocks until you feel a stretch in the front of your thigh. Hold the strech, then roll over to your left side and repeat with your right leg.

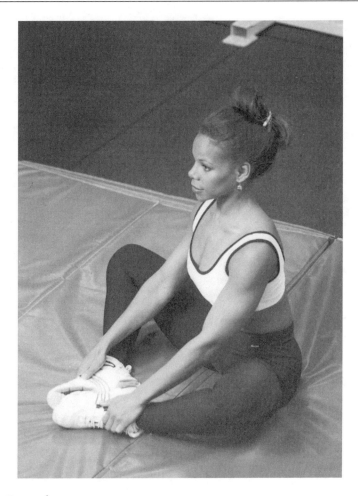

Groin Stretch

1. Sit on the floor with your legs bent and the soles of your feet together. Place your hands on your feet, and press your upper body forward until you feel a stretch in the inside of your upper thighs. Keep your back straight throughout this stretch. Relax by returning to an upright position.

Calf Stretch

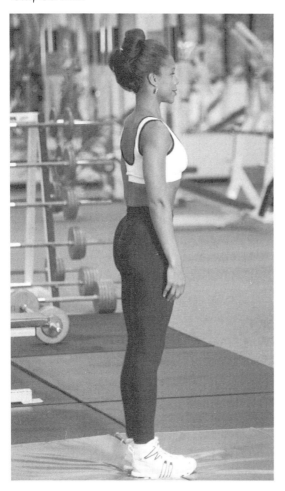 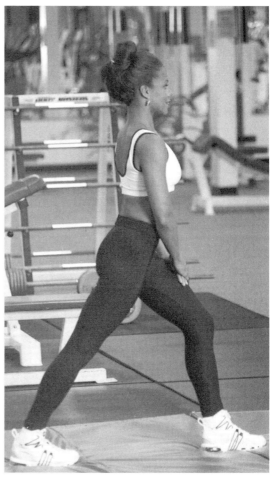

1. Stand tall with your abdominals contracted, your chest lifted, and your shoulders relaxed.

2. Lunge backward with your right foot, and press your heel down until you feel a stretch in your right calf. (To get a good stretch, keep the toes of both feet pointed forward.) Hold the stretch, then switch legs and repeat.

Shoulder Stretch

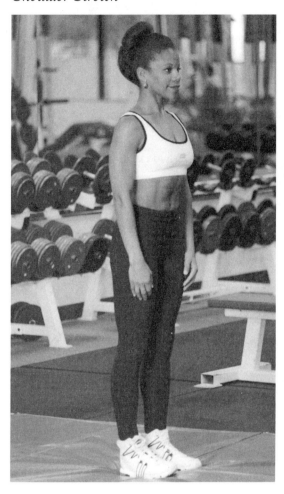 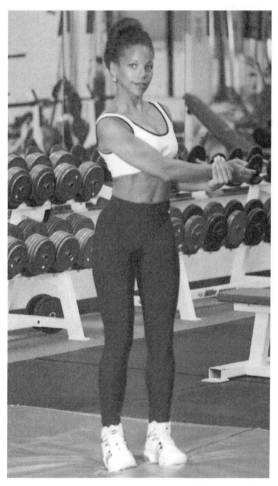

1. Stand with your feet hip width apart, your abdominals contracted, and your arms resting at your sides.

2. Grab your right arm with your left hand. Keeping your shoulders down and your hips square to the front, pull your right arm across to the left side of your body (your right elbow should be slightly bent). Hold the stretch, then repeat on the other arm.

Back Stretch

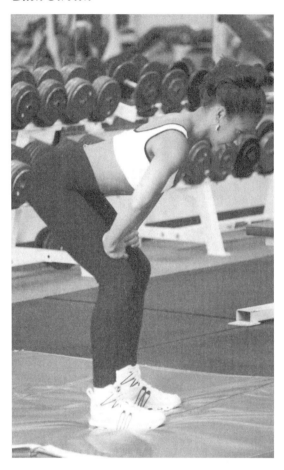 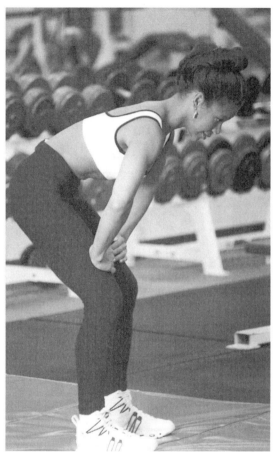

1. Stand with your feet shoulder-width apart. Keeping your back straight, bend forward and place your hands on your upper thighs.

2. Contract your abdominals and round your back until you feel a nice stretch. Hold and repeat.

Neck Stretch

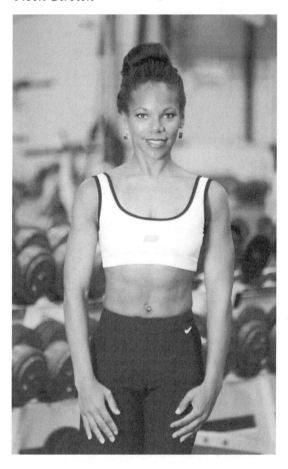 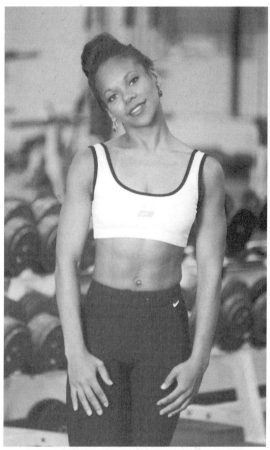

1. Stand tall with your feet apart, your knees bent, and your hands resting on your thighs.

2. Tilt your head to the right and hold it, then tilt it to the left and hold it. Repeat.

Fitness While You Travel

Although many of us view traveling as an excuse to take a vacation from everything—including our fitness regimen—it's really important to keep up your program when you're on the road. Naturally, you can't do *everything* you'd do at home in a hotel, but taking time to work out while you travel will keep you healthy and will give you more energy for the things you want to do on your trip, be it an all-day sightseeing excursion or leading a weekend business seminar. (And yes, you *can* count that long walk on the beach at sunset as part of your cardio routine!)

Unfortunately, trying to maintain a fitness program while you're traveling can be a real pain. Unfamiliar surroundings, inconveniently located health clubs, and precious little time are some of the many pitfalls facing us when we go on the road. I spend a large part of my time traveling, speaking at conventions,

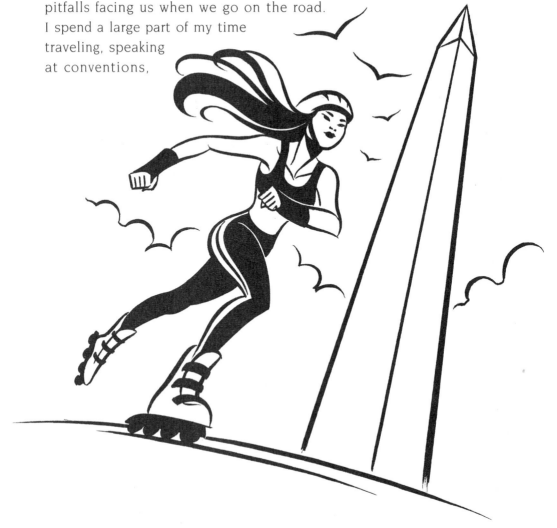

leading seminars, and making public appearances, and I always try to work out so I don't miss a beat. Over time, I've developed a system that works for me.

First of all, I don't worry about skipping a workout or following the same program I do when I'm at home. In fact, by cutting back on my workouts, I avoid getting sick or injured from adding the stress of exercising to the stress of travel. If I try to keep my level of activity the same as at home, I just get burned out. Instead, I make being on the road work to my advantage. I've discovered that travel can actually be a fitness buff's best friend: it provides a great opportunity to vary your routine and helps keep you from falling into a rut. Keep the following points in mind when travelling:

- ◆ Listen to your body. If you're too tired to exercise, don't.

- ◆ If you can't find the time to do some structured exercise, combine your daily activities with some fitness. Walk to your meeting or to dinner, and use the stairs instead of the elevator.

- ◆ When I travel to a new city, I like to in-line skate, jog, or walk around and take in the local sights, which helps stimulate my mind as well as my heart and lungs.

- ◆ Properly timed periods of physical activity will help keep your body on track. Working out right after you arrive can help combat any jet lag, and working out in the late afternoon can help ensure a good night's sleep.

- ◆ If you're flying to your destination, the United States Olympic Committee suggests that you drink plenty of liquids before, during, and after the flight, since airplane cabins are very dry. Bring a supply of bottled water with you when traveling (increased water consumption can also help prevent jet lag).

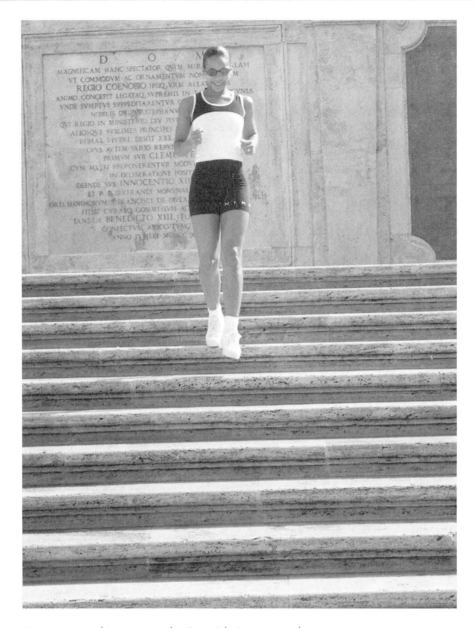

Here I am working out on the Spanish Steps in Italy.

◆ Try to use the time during your plane ride to relax, listen to music, read a book, or practice your visualization and meditation techniques. De-stressing plays a big part in staying healthy—mentally and physically.

◆ Sitting for long periods of time can cause your body to become stiff because blood "pools" (or settles) in your lower body. Get up and walk around the cabin every hour or so, and use the office stretches from chapter 3 to help keep your muscles loose. Some airlines are now playing in-flight exercise videos, which is a great idea! I can't tell you how many times I have seen people plant themselves in their seat for an entire five-hour flight and never get up. Do your body a favor and make a point of moving around.

In addition, you should allow one day of reduced training for every time zone you cross, especially when traveling from the West Coast to the East Coast. It helps to book your flights so that you will be arriving during daylight hours, since sunlight helps regulate your biological clock. When planning your trip, just remember this basic rule: if you're flying west, you want to leave later in the day, and if you are traveling east, fly out earlier in the morning (if your schedule permits).

Fitness on the Go

I've developed a resistive routine that you can perform with lightweight rubber exercise bands called the Xertube—found at most sporting goods stores, or see the Resources section at the end of this book—to enable you to do your strength training wherever you go. Just take the tubing out of your suitcase, work out, and throw it back into your luggage when you're done. Start your workout by marching around the room for several minutes. Then stretch your muscles so you're ready to get busy. For a mini cardio workout, do like I do and whip out your jump rope. Do one set of eight to twelve reps for each exercise.

Leg Extension (works the quadriceps)

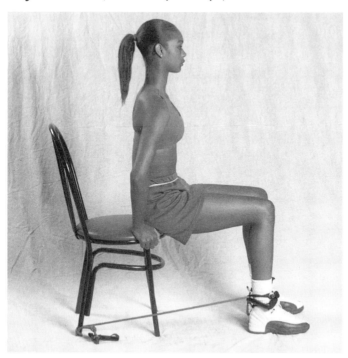

1. Sit on a chair with your knees bent, feet flat on the floor, and abdominals contracted. Wrap one end of the Xertube around the back leg of the chair and secure it underneath. Tie the other end around your right ankle. Make sure that there's not a lot of slack in the tubing, so that it's a challenge to straighten your leg.

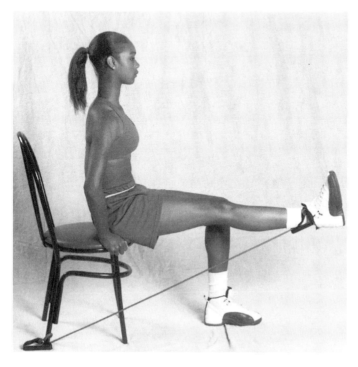

2. While maintaining your body position, straighten your right leg to hip height, keeping your foot flexed. Return to the starting position and complete reps. Repeat on the other leg.

Leg Curl (works the hamstrings)

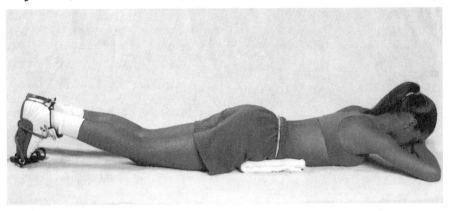

1. Tie the Xertube into a small loop (to increase resistance), then slip the tube around your left ankle and over the arch of your right foot. Lie facedown on the floor with your head supported on your forearms. Place a towel or pillow under your hips so that your legs are elevated off the floor. Tilt your pelvis and contract your abdominals.

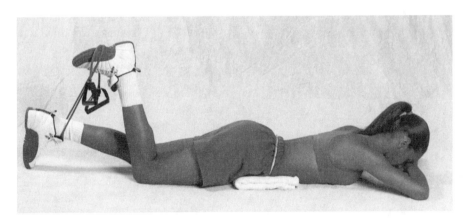

2. Tighten your buttocks and curl your right heel toward your glutes. Straighten your leg back out and return to the starting position. Do all reps, then switch to the opposite leg and repeat.

***Seated* Row** (works the rhomboids, trapezius, posterior deltoids, and biceps)

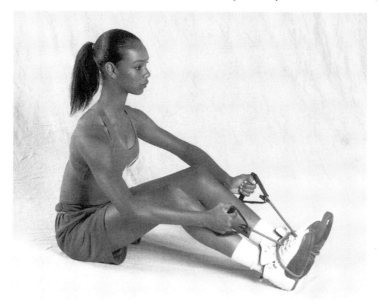

1. Sit on the floor with your legs extended in front of you and your knees slightly bent. Wrap the tube around the insteps of both feet, and tie it on top for stability. Grasp the handles of the rubber tubing in both hands with your palms facing each other. Continue to lean slightly forward with your arms outstretched toward your toes and your elbows slightly bent, keeping your back straight.

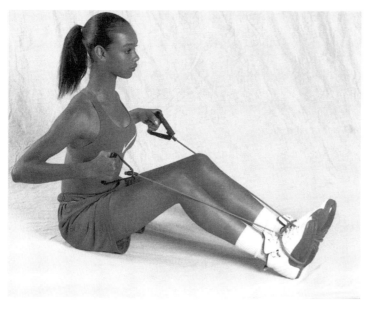

2. Squeeze your shoulder blades together and pull the handles towards your torso until your hands touch your sides. Pause and return to the starting position.

Standing Chest Press (works the pectorals)

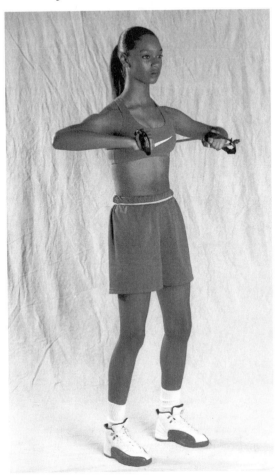 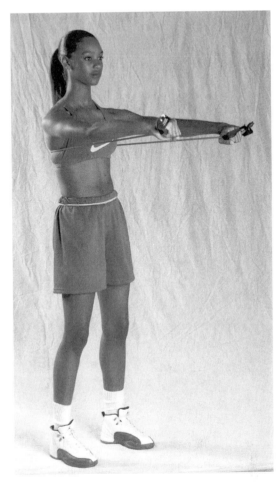

1. Stand with your feet shoulder-width apart, knees slightly bent. Abdominals should be contracted, the rib cage lifted, with your tailbone pointing toward the floor. Place the Xertube around your back and under your arms. Wrap the tube around your hands with your palms facing down, elbows at shoulder height.

2. Squeeze your shoulder blades together and push the tube out in front of your body. Return to the starting position.

Lateral Raise (works the deltoids)

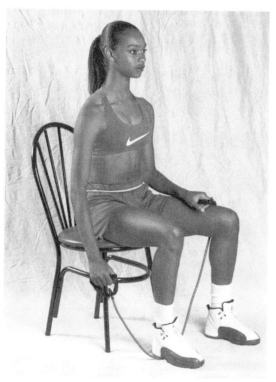 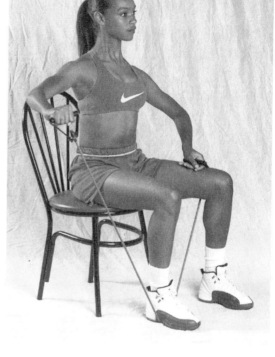

1. Sit on a chair and place your right foot on the center of the tube. Hold one handle in your left hand, and rest this hand on your left thigh. (You can control the amount of resistance you apply with this hand while supporting your upper body.) Grasp the other handle with your right hand, palm facing in, your arm extended toward your foot.

2. Lift your right arm up and out, away from your body. Once your hand reaches shoulder height, pause, then return to the starting position. Complete all reps then switch to the other side.

Overhead Tricep Extension (works the triceps)

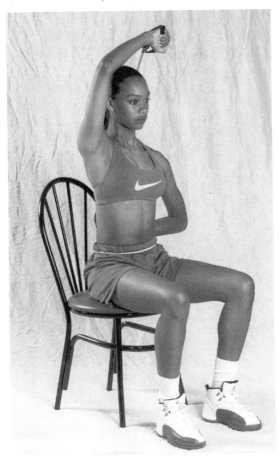
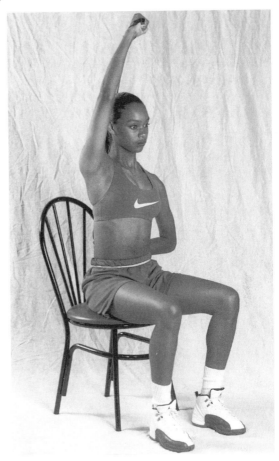

1. Sit tall in a chair with your feet flat on the floor. Hold one end of the rubber tube (not the handle) with your left hand anchored against your lower back, palm facing out and thumb up. Grasp the handle at the other end of the tube with your hand resting near the back of your head, thumb facing down and elbow pointed towards the ceiling.

2. Straighten your right arm, pulling the tube upward. Pause and return to the starting position. Perform all reps, then repeat on the other side.

Seated Bicep Curl (works the biceps)

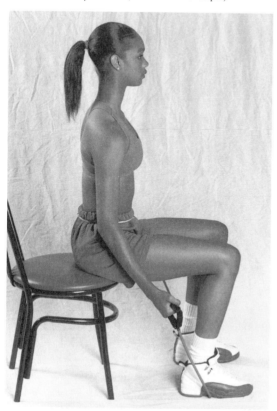 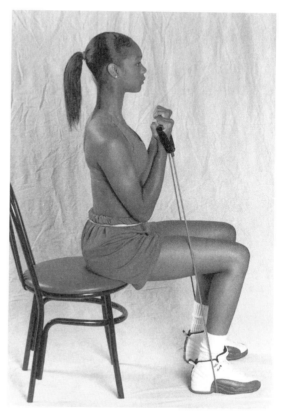

1. Sit on the edge of a chair with your legs shoulder width apart. Place the Xertube underneath your feet, and hold a handle in each hand, with your arms extended down toward the floor.

2. Keeping your elbows close to your sides and your wrists in line with your forearms, curl your palms toward your shoulders. Pause and return to the starting position.

Crunch with a Twist (works the rectus abdominis and external obliques)

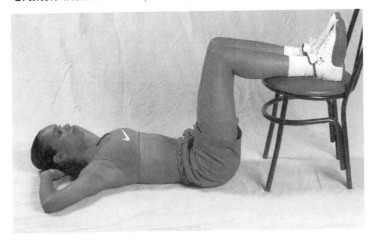

1. Lie with your back on the floor. Put your heels up on a chair seat so that your knees are directly over your hips. Place one thumb behind each ear— fingertips touching but not clasped—with your elbows open.

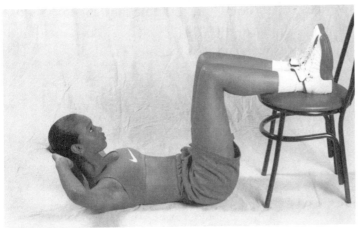

2. Exhale and lift your head, neck, and shoulders off the floor, as you would for a regular crunch.

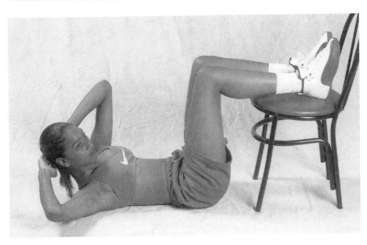

3. Rotate your torso toward your right knee, leading with your left shoulder without moving your hips. Return to the center position, with your torso still lifted off the ground, and rotate toward your left knee, leading with your right shoulder. Return to the starting position. Repeat for fifteen to twenty reps.

When using the Xertube, it's important to use smooth, controlled movements throughout the full range of motion. Don't jerk the band; try to keep your movements fluid. Maintain tension on the band from start to finish while always making sure that the band is securely fastened before you begin each exercise. It's also helpful to periodically check your tube for signs of wear, just in case it needs to be replaced.

An Automobile Program

The following exercises are great to use when you're traveling by car—and they're perfect for people who get tense while sitting in traffic on a crowded freeway. (I know I have several friends who lose it whenever they have to drive in rush hour traffic. You know the people I mean—those horn-blowing finger-givers.) By doing these simple movements, you can relieve some of the tension caused by stressing out in traffic, or by spending too many hours sitting behind the wheel.

Steering Wheel Squeeze

To help relieve tension in your hands and forearms, grip your steering wheel, using the standard ten o'clock and two o'clock driving positions and squeeze tightly for four or five seconds. Release.

Shoulder Blade Squeeze

Many people have a tendency to "round" their shoulders while they drive. To help correct this poor posture, squeeze your shoulder blades together as you lift your rib cage. Hold the "squeeze" for ten seconds and relax.

Abdominal Tightener

This exercise should be used in combination with the shoulder blade squeeze to combat another form of bad posture—slouching down in the seat. Begin by making sure that you are sitting up straight, with your buttocks and lower back pressed firmly into the seat. Contract your abdominals while adding in the shoulder blade squeeze, and hold for five seconds. Release your abdominals, then return to the relaxed erect starting position.

　　Just like in the office, shoulder shrugs, head rolls, and wrist bends can be done for some added relaxation. The goal is to release the tension that has built up in the various parts of your body. It's about reducing stress and feeling your best.

5

Exercise for
Everybody

Exercise and Pregnancy

One question I get asked a lot is "What type of exercise should I do while I'm pregnant?" When you're exercising for two, the first thing you want to do is check with your doctor. In 1994, the American College of Obstetricians and Gynecologists (ACOG) established some new guidelines for exercise in pregnancy and postpartum .

Currently, there is no data available that would indicate that pregnant women should limit the amount of exercise they do. For women who do not have any additional risk factors that could cause adverse maternal or perinatal complications, ACOG recommends the following:

♦ During pregnancy, women can continue to exercise. Health benefits can be derived even from mild to moderate exercise routines. Regular exercise (at least three times per week) is preferable to intermittent activity.

♦ Women should avoid exercise in the supine position (flat on the back) after the first trimester. Such a position is associated with decreased cardiac output in most pregnant women, since oxygen is diverted away from the uterus—to the muscles you're working—during vigorous exercise. Such exercises are best avoided during pregnancy. Prolonged periods of motionless standing should also be avoided.

◆ Women should be aware of the decreased oxygen available for aerobic exercise during pregnancy. They should be encouraged to modify the intensity of their exercise according to maternal symptoms. Pregnant women should stop exercising when fatigued and *never* exercise to exhaustion. Weight-bearing exercises may, under some circumstances, be continued at intensities similar to those prior to pregnancy. Non-weight-bearing exercises, such as cycling or swimming, will minimize the risk of injury and facilitate the continuation of exercise during pregnancy.

◆ Weight gain during pregnancy should serve as a guide to the types of exercises performed. The extra weight can throw off your sense of balance and be detrimental to maternal or fetal well-being, especially during the third trimester. Any types of exercise involving the potential for even mild abdominal trauma should be strictly avoided. (In other words: no mountain biking or snowboarding.)

◆ Pregnancy requires an additional three hundred calories a day in order to maintain metabolic homeostasis. Women who exercise during pregnancy should be particularly careful to ensure that they're eating enough food.

◆ Pregnant women who exercise in the first trimester should enhance their bodies' cooling mechanism by having adequate hydration, appropriate clothing, and an optimal environmental surrounding during exercise.

◆ Many of the physiologic and morphologic (body weight) changes persist four to six weeks postpartum. Prepregnancy exercise routines should, therefore, be resumed gradually, based on a woman's capability.

There are also several factors that your obstetrician would consider contraindications for exercise during pregnancy (which means you should lay off exercising until the blessed event, so take a break and just chill). They include:

◆ Pregnancy-induced hypertension

◆ Preterm rupture of membrane

◆ Preterm labor during the prior or current pregnancy

◆ Incompetent cervix

◆ Persistent second- to third-trimester bleeding

◆ Intrauterine growth retardation

Now, you know how much your body changes during pregnancy. It's important to reestablish healthy habits—eating right and exercising—as soon as possible, so that you can regain your muscle tone and lose those unwanted extra pounds. Don't allow too much time to pass, 'cause your muscles will start to sag, and that'll just give you the blues. Besides, a well-designed workout program will not only help you tone up, improve your circulation, promote healing of the abdominal muscles, and reduce the risk of back problems—a concern of every toddler-toting mom—it will also give you the energy you need to keep up with your little dumpling.

Fitness for Older Adults

Did you know that by the year 2030 one in five Americans will be over sixty-five years old? Older adults face numerous problems as they mature, many of which are associated with decreased levels of activity. For various reasons, people just stop being active as they get older. Cutting back on the amount of physical activity you do can intensify the aging process and also make you susceptible to the following:

◆ An increased risk of heart disease

◆ A higher incidence of osteoporosis

◆ Increased difficulties with arthritis

◆ A higher incidence of falls

◆ Trouble maintaining "ideal" body weight

What can you do to make your golden years healthier? <u>EXERCISE!</u> People who maintain an active lifestyle live longer and have fewer health problems than those who don't. It also helps them improve their quality of life, to boot. Major benefits of a fitness program include:

◆ Lower blood pressure and cholesterol

◆ Increased bone density (thicker bones)

◆ Increased strength and stamina

◆ Increased self esteem and confidence

◆ Better balance and coordination

◆ Lower levels of body fat

As with anyone beginning an exercise program, it's important for more mature adults to get the approval of a physician before starting out. This step is especially critical in ensuring that your program is safe and effective. Many older adults take various medications to treat their health conditions, and those drugs can change the person's response to exercise. For example, some heart medications, such as beta blockers, can suppress your heart rate during exercise, making your training heart rate lower than someone not on medication (meaning you may overexert yourself). Other medications can make you feel light headed, too tired to exercise, or cause muscle cramps.

Just like anyone else, an older adult is limited by the current condition of his or her health and well-being. Common problems for the elderly, such as arthritis (which includes osteoarthritis), deterioration of cartilage in the joints (such as the knees), and rheumatoid arthritis (an inflammation that can affect many different joints, including the hands), all make it difficult to perform even the simplest of movements.

Osteoporosis is another common problem for people over sixty-five. Osteoporosis is caused by a gradual loss of bone mineral density, which weakens the bones, making them brittle and more susceptible to fracture and breakage. Osteoporosis is brought on by a calcium deficiency and aging. Fortunately, this degenerative disease can be treated with a calcium-rich diet and weight-bearing exercises (anything from walking to tennis), which help increase bone density and maintain elasticity. In addition, older people who increase their level of activity often experience improvements in balance, strength, coordination, and flexibility, all of which help prevent falls that can result in a debilitating fracture.

One of my clients, whom I love and adore, was as fragile as a china teacup when we first began working together seven years ago. It seemed as if she had an osteoporosis-related fracture—rib, ankle, wrist—almost every month. But after designing a program for her that included low-impact and water aerobics, walking, strength training, and stretching, she's now as strong as a bull. At seventy, she boogies down on the dance floor whenever she gets the chance—and I can't remember the last time she had an injury. I feel proud when I see my friend walking tall and getting a bang out of life!

Many mature adults suffer from depression, low self-esteem, and feelings of isolation, which can all affect overall health, as well as the person's willingness to participate in an exercise program. Get yourself checked out, and then get moving. Check out chapter 3 for more tips on getting started and for my senior-friendly GetFit program.

Finding a Program in Your Community

As discussed earlier, one of the most important factors in any exercise program is social support, for young and old people alike. Interacting with other people your own age while exercising is a great way to stay motivated, and it will definitely help you stick with your program (it's also a *great* way to make new friends). Check the resources available in your area to locate a program that uses a combination of exercises such as t'ai chi (which has been shown to reduce the incidence of falls among older adults), yoga, water exercises, walking, swimming, ballroom dancing, and weight training, along with social activities that are specifically designed to promote the health of older adults. The best places to look for these types of programs are YMCAs, community centers, local universities, and hospitals. Many of them offer programs at reduced fees for adults sixty years of age and older, and some may even allow you to participate for free, or on a "scholarship."

Exercise for the Overweight

If you are clinically overweight (more than 20 percent above what should be your healthy body weight) and want to participate in an exercise program, you need to take some basic precautions to ensure that your experience will be a safe one. The most important thing to do is to get your physician's approval for beginning a program. Let him or her know what you will be doing during your workouts. If you have ever experienced any breathlessness, pain, or persistent discomfort, be sure to report it to your doctor.

During the program itself, follow all the guidelines I laid out in this section of the book and in chapters 2 and 3. Exercise in a slow, moderate manner, using good form and alignment. The extra weight you're carrying puts an added strain on your body as you move, making even moderate activity, such as walking up the stairs, difficult. It is also important that you concentrate on your breathing, since excess fat can adversely affect how you breathe, causing you to get winded easily. Finally, stay hydrated—overweight people tend to have problems dissipating body heat.

If you feel uncomfortable exercising in public, follow the home or office program of daily activities outlined in chapters 2 and 3. They should help get you started, plus the stop-and-go nature of the programs will allow you to spread your activity out over the entire day without leading to overexertion. Once you feel more comfortable exercising, go out and hit the road!

Most importantly, remember that it helps to keep a good mental attitude and just do your thing. Keep moving forward, and you'll reach your goals.

6

Sneakers and Trainers and Gyms (Oh My!)

Rain, Rain, Go Away! (Exercise and the Environment)

One of these days you may find yourself exercising outside, in a less-than-favorable environment. Knowing just what to do in bad weather could mean more to you than being comfortable—it could save your life. Exercising in really hot weather can produce heat-related illnesses, such as heat exhaustion or heat stroke, and in extreme cases, death. Both of these problems can be traced to dehydration, a loss of bodily fluids caused by not drinking enough liquids before, during, and after exercise. During the warm summer months, the body's ability to cool itself is made more difficult by the heat and humidity. Humidity makes it harder for the sweat to evaporate into the already moist air.

Hot Weather

One way to help you get the most out of your workout in the heat is to slowly acclimate to the stress that will affect your body when you exercise in hot weather. Several weeks of moderate exercise in the heat will produce desirable changes such as a lower body temperature and an increased rate of sweating. (Basically, this means that your body is learning to adjust to the heat and is cooling itself more efficiently.) You know how an air conditioner sometimes takes a while to adjust before it starts pumping out the cool air? Well, your body is no different.

Another way to prevent problems in the heat is to work out either early or late in the day, avoiding the extreme heat of midmorning and early afternoon hours. Wear loose-fitting, cotton clothing in light colors to help promote heat loss. Although dark colors may be fashionable and slimming, they also absorb more heat than lighter ones.

It's also critical that you get a head start on replacing the fluids you'll lose through exercise. Drink at least fifteen to twenty ounces of liquid about twenty minutes prior to working out and continue to drink eight ounces every fifteen minutes during prolonged bouts of exercise.

If you experience any of the warnings signs of heat-related illness— such as "goose bumps" on the upper chest and arms, chills, throbbing pressure in the head, unsteadiness, nausea, or dry skin— stop immediately and find someplace cool to rest. Beating the heat is definitely a case where an ounce of prevention is worth a pound of cure.

Cold Weather

Although exercising in cold weather may seem a little less intimidating, it shouldn't be taken lightly. Believe it or not, proper hydration may be even more important when it's cold out. Although the air is cooler, it's also drier—due to low humidity—so moisture is quickly absorbed off the body as it evaporates. This may cause dehydration. Follow the same guidelines that you would for hot weather, drinking eight ounces of liquid every fifteen minutes.

Just as in warm weather, proper clothing can make a big difference. During the winter, it's best to dress in several different layers of clothing so that you stay both warm and dry. When it's cold outside, it's important to wear clothes close to your skin that are made of materials such as polypropylene, which wicks away sweat and doesn't absorb perspiration the way cotton does. For an outer layer, materials such as Gore-Tex are great. They help repel moisture while allowing the body to cool itself. Regardless of what you're wearing, though, if you're already warm when you leave the house, you probably have on too much clothing. Still, there are a few pieces of clothing that you definitely cannot do without: a hat and gloves are musts. You lose most of your body heat through you head and hands, so be smart and dress the part.

Getting Off on the Right Foot

There is another essential piece of fitness equipment that you can't do without: good shoes. Choosing your athletic footwear can be confusing these days, with all the different styles and brands that are available. How do you know if you are getting your money's worth? If you follow Miss Donna's simple guidelines, you simply can't go wrong.

◆ Pick the shoe to fit your activity. If you're a runner, don't use a shoe made for tennis. Shoe manufacturers design shoes to meet the specific demands of each individual activity. Sneakers designed for sports that require lots of lateral movement, such as tennis, are made to provide more support in the sides of the shoe. Sneakers designed for sports such as running need to absorb the impact caused while moving forward and are, therefore, made with more cushioning both in the heel and the front of the shoe. If you do several different activities and don't want to spend a fortune on several pairs of sneakers, consider cross-trainers, which are specifically designed for a variety of different types of exercise.

◆ If you are tall and heavy, choose a shoe made with a dense midsole, such as a polyurethane material. People who are smaller can wear a lighter shoe made with a compression-molded ethyl vinyl acetane or EVA midsole.

◆ Proper shoe selection is also important for preventing injuries. If you suffer from knee pain, pick a shoe with a firm sole that helps control motion and provides stability. A "straight last" shoe is your best bet if you are a pronator (your foot rolls to the inside), since the straighter the shoe, the more medial (inside) support it has.

◆ When you go to buy your new shoes, bring the type of socks you plan to wear while exercising. This will help ensure a proper fit. It's also important to shop in the afternoon, since the size of your feet increases during the day. Try on different brands to get a good feel for which shoes are more comfortable on your feet, and take them for a spin around the store.

◆ Finally, your training shoes should be replaced about every four to six months. Looking at the outer sole is usually not a good way to tell if the shoe is worn, since the midsole inside the shoe loses its shock-absorbing properties long before the bottom wears out.

Take it from Miss D: follow these rules, and you'll always be putting your best foot forward.

Joining a Club

One of your goals might be to join a health club, a community recreation center, or the local Y. In case you're confused about which ones are the best, here are some questions to ask yourself, along with a few tips that you might find useful in selecting the gym that's right for you.

The Facility

◆ Is it clean and well maintained? Is the upholstery torn, the weight equipment rusted or in need of repair? Is the carpeting frayed or dirty, and are the rest rooms and showers clean? If you don't like the answers to any of these questions, then run— don't walk—to the nearest exit.

◆ Does it provide a variety of programs? Is there a good selection of aerobic classes, lots of fitness equipment (cardiovascular and strength training), day care, specialty programs such as boxaerobics, spinning, or kickboxing, and sports programs like basketball and squash? The more a club has to offer, the more likely you'll be to stick with it for the long haul.

◆ Is it close to home or work? Remember, convenience is a major factor in being able to stick with an exercise program.

◆ Do you like the members? If the other members make you feel uncomfortable, you'll be less likely to go work out.

◆ Is the facility crowded during the times when you wish to use it? Are there lines for the pieces of equipment you want to use? To get a good feel for the club, it helps to plan a visit at the times you are going to work out .

The Staff

◆ Do they have a degree in the field? An education in the area of health, physical education, or a similar area is essential to the safety and effectiveness of a member's program.

◆ Are they certified? A certified fitness professional is someone who has met a specific standard within the industry that will help ensure the quality of the program. The American Council on Exercise (ACE) and ACSM are two well-respected certification organizations.

◆ Do they provide a screening and orientation process? These procedures will aid the fitness staff at the club in designing an individualized program that will be more successful.

◆ Are they friendly and motivational? A good instructor can make all the difference in the world when it comes to achieving your fitness goals. A bad one, on the other hand, can totally turn you off to exercise.

The Agreement

◆ Are the terms of the contract clearly defined? Are all the options, such as payment plans and levels of membership, spelled out, including any previous verbal agreements?

◆ Have there been any complaints filed against the club? Check with the Better Business Bureau to see if the club has had any problems in the last few years.

◆ Can you try out the facility before joining? Some clubs will give you a free pass to come work out before you sign the contract.

◆ Are there provisions if you move, or if you quit the club? Can your membership be bought or transferred, or will you be stuck with a membership you can't use?

Finding a Personal Trainer

Whether you work out at home or at the gym, a personal trainer can be just the motivator you need. Although you now know how to make educated decisions regarding your fitness future, it still helps to get some feedback on how it's going. Even fitness professionals such as myself benefit from an extra set of eyes from time to time. Choosing a personal trainer is a lot like choosing any other type of specialist; you want to get the most qualified person that you can.

First of all, it's helpful if your potential trainer has a background in exercise science or exercise physiology. A formal education in one of these areas means your trainer will be able to design a program that incorporates both aerobic and anaerobic components for optimum results. It's also preferable if your trainer has met some sort of standard of professional competency within the field. ACE offers a certification for personal trainers that is considered one of the best in the industry.

The National Strength and Conditioning Association offers a certificate for a Certified Strength and Conditioning Specialist (C.S.C.S.). This credential demonstrates that your trainer has the knowledge required to design and administer conditioning programs. This is important, since a good training program requires the proper "cycling" of all of the various components of your schedule: aerobic and anaerobic conditioning, strength training, and flexibility. (Other organizations that certify fitness professionals include the Aerobics and Fitness Association of American (AFAA) and the National Academy of Sports Medicine.)

Finally, there are several specialty certifications through organizations like the American College of Sports Medicine (ACSM), that offer a Health Fitness Instructor certification. This covers important areas such as fitness testing and exercise prescription.

It's essential that your trainer have a thorough working knowledge of how to handle medical emergencies, CPR and first aid training included. They should also have liability insurance, in case you get injured due to negligence on the part of your trainer.

The question of cost could also influence your decision. Does the trainer have clear-cut billing procedures and cancellation policies that he or she puts in writing? Most trainers charge between $25 to $100 per hour, so price could also be a consideration.

The best thing you can do after all is said and done is to meet your prospective trainer and see how well you mesh. Ask for references from other clients they've trained. After taking all of this information into account, you should have no problem making an educated decision.

Fitness Testing

Before you begin a structured exercise program, it's a good idea to get a fitness evaluation. Such an assessment measures all of the components of fitness in an effort to find your strengths and weaknesses. This information can then be used to design an effective individualized exercise program. A fitness assessment can also be used after you've already started an exercise program to evaluate your progress, and it can help motivate and educate you. Here are some of the tests that should be performed as part of a comprehensive fitness evaluation:

Cardiorespiratory endurance. Measured while you pedal a stationary bike, or walk on a treadmill. Your heart rate is recorded throughout the test and is used to determine the efficiency of your heart and lungs during exercise. Your blood pressure is also monitored during the test to watch for any potential problems.

Muscular strength. Your level of strength is normally determined using a handgrip dynamometer, a device specifically designed for this purpose. It involves performing an isometric contraction that requires little or no movement of the hand, wrist, and forearm muscles.

Muscular endurance. Determined by the number of sit-ups performed for a one-minute time period, and the total number of push-ups done in an unlimited time.

Flexibility. Assessed by using a test known as the "sit and reach," which is essentially an indication of your ability to touch your toes. This tests the flexibility of your lower back and the hamstrings on the back of your thighs.

Body composition. Estimates the amount of fat under the skin. It's sort of an advanced version of the "pinch an inch" test. Using calipers, skinfold measurements are taken at various sites on the body to determine your percentage of body fat.

These tests should be performed by qualified personnel at your health club, local hospital, or university. Just call and ask if they do fitness evaluations for the public so that you can use the results in designing your exercise program. When the test is completed, you should get a printout that tells you how you did in each one of these areas. Your fitness instructor or personal trainer can then use the data to help you set realistic goals for your exercise program.

Exercise and Injury

Have you ever been in the middle of your exercise routine and suddenly felt pain where there had been none? You might not have known whether to continue or to stop. Learning to distinguish between the discomfort of a hard workout and the pain of a potential injury is not an easy skill to master, but it's something that can't be overlooked by anyone who works out. Ignoring tight, sore muscles could lead to something far worse than poor workouts—it could result in an injury.

There are several simple ways to determine if an injury is minor (and worth ignoring), such as a tight muscle that loosens up as you exercise, or if it's more serious and requires medical attention (such as a pulled or sprained muscle). First of all, if a pain starts early in your workout and continues throughout, it might indicate a problem. Also, if you have pain at the end of your training session and it persists into the next day, it could be a sign of possible trouble. Another sure sign of injury is swelling of the affected area. Check to see if it is red, puffy, or warm to the touch. In addition, use stretching as a tool to distinguish between the pain of an injury and the everyday effects of a hard workout. If the pain lessens with stretching, it's probably the type brought on by muscle damage caused during hard exercise. This is just the normal delayed onset muscle soreness that is typical of any strenuous physical activity. If not...uh-oh!

As I've already mentioned, physical activity helps increase awareness. Learn to listen to your body. Hopefully, the next time you're exercising and feel a twinge, you'll be better equipped to make an informed decision. Remember: listen to your body. It tells it like it is.

Treatment of Sports Injuries

If an injury does occur, take appropriate action by seeking medical help as soon as possible. Many people avoid getting treatment, hoping the condition will get better on its own. Often this can make the problem even worse. Until medical help arrives, there are a few things to do immediately. Remember this simple formula: RICE (Rest, Ice,

Compression, and Elevation). All of these steps are designed to help reduce the swelling brought on by an injury, which is an important component of getting back on your feet (so to speak), as soon as possible. If you sprained your ankle playing softball, you would use an elastic bandage to wrap the affected area in ice, keeping your leg propped up. I'd advise laying low for a few days. Another helpful hint? Never put heat on an affected area during the first forty-eight to seventy-two hours; it can aggravate an injury. If you follow these simple steps, you'll have an enjoyable, injury-free workout. And keeping you up and running is what it's all about, right?

7

Child's Play

When I was growing up in Silver Spring, Maryland, I began participating in sports at an early age. By the time I was five I was a baton girl, and in the years that followed I took up swimming, dance, softball, track and field, gymnastics, and cheerleading. Whenever I picked up a new activity, I became totally focused on it. I loved training for an event, the challenge of competing, and the satisfaction that came when I actually won. More than anything else, I loved the way athletics made me feel: self-assured, confident, and strong. Playing sports might have been mentally and physically challenging, but it was also about having fun and sharing my experiences with my family and friends. The sense of pride that I obtained from participating in sports and dance—from my parents, coaches, and teachers telling me to believe I could achieve whatever I set my mind to, if I worked hard enough—has stayed with me throughout my adult life. It's gone a long way toward making me who I am today.

One of the most important lessons I learned during those formative years was that losing is not necessarily a bad thing. When you participate in competitive sports you don't always win, but you quickly learn that failure is an inevitable part of success. You deal with it and move on to the next challenge.

These lessons have been so instrumental in shaping my life that for the past eight years I've been working to get the message across to those who need to hear it most—today's youth. I'm very involved with the Boys & Girls Club of America and Nike's P.L.A.Y. (Participate in the Lives of America's Youth) program; I also give motivational speeches at schools around the world as part of my own StayFit Kids program. My program is aimed at instilling the virtues of a healthy, educational, and drug-free lifestyle in kids from all walks of life. Through the years, the kids I've worked with have ended up teaching me a thing or two about life as well.

For instance, two years ago, I was invited to visit a Boys & Girls Club in Chicago's inner city, along with several of my colleagues, to speak with kids and lead them through a physical activity session. Unfortunately, I was not able to attend the program due to a prior engagement, but I arranged to visit the club the next day to lead a seminar.

When I arrived in Chicago the evening after the first event had ended, my colleagues filled my ears with horror stories about their visit at the B&G Club. They told me that the kids were rude and disobedient—totally out of control. My colleagues vowed that they would *never* go back to this club again. This worried me because several of the kids were supposed to assist me in teaching a class to four hundred fitness professionals the following evening. The event was aimed at getting my peers excited about volunteering their time and energy to help underprivileged kids. I woke up the next morning feeling jittery and unsure about what would take place that night. Over the years, I'd visited many B&G Clubs and community centers around the country and planned hundreds of events just like the one we would be doing that evening. The experience had always been rewarding, and a lot of fun. After hearing my colleagues' horror stories, I kept asking myself, "Why should this time be any different? What's up with these kids? "

The kids arrived an hour and a half before the event. I introduced myself, reviewed the purpose of the event, and explained the rules of play. I asked if everyone felt they could comply with my rules; everyone responded affirmatively. I spoke about our game plan, asked for suggestions, and then gave them their assignments and teamed them up with my various colleagues—some of whom were the same folks who'd had such a bad experience with these kids a couple of days before.

The event started with the usual chatter, but then it was "prime time" as the kids, my colleagues, and fitness pros from the Midwest all got busy. The class was set up like an obstacle course, or what we fitness people refer to as a "circuit" class. There were eight stations. Each group performed an exercise at each station for one minute, doing various activities such as the Suicide Run, the Basketball Shuffle, or some good old-fashioned push-ups.

The evening was "all that, and a bag of chips," as the kids like to say. (Translation for those of you over forty: it was *way* cool.) Throughout the program, the kids were professional, motivated, and well behaved—not exactly what I'd been expecting. After the event was over, many of the instructors inquired as to how they could start volunteering their services and start programs in their own communities. Mission accomplished!

Afterward, we took the kids to dinner. They were so excited about the event that they kept asking us when were we going to do it again. Being just as excited as they were, I made a commitment to visit their club during my next visit to Chicago. (And yes, I've been back to visit them several times since then.)

This experience was a real eye-opener for me. It reminded me not to judge people based on other folks' opinions, and not to give up on young kids. When I met with the kids, I told them exactly what I expected of them, and I let them know that I believed that we would succeed. It's all about respecting each other and learning to work together as a team. I've learned that kids need love, respect, and support. Sometimes—as in the story I just told you—what they need most is to be given high standards to live up to. Time and time again, I've found that kids will abide by the rules you lay out for them. If you expect them to give you their best, you have to give them your best in return—ain't no half-steppin'. The most important thing you can teach a child is that respect isn't given automatically. It's something you have to earn. My goal in working with kids is to teach them the skills and tools they need to develop their self-confidence and sense of self-worth. Once they learn to respect themselves, they'll respect others as well.

Unfortunately, many kids growing up nowadays don't have the

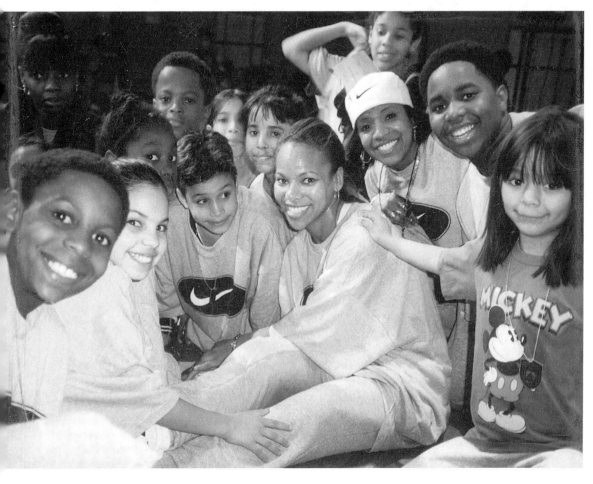

...with "my" kids

love, support and opportunites that I have had. To add to this, kids are becoming a second generation of couch potatoes. According to the National Health and Nutrition Examination Survey (NHANES-III), released in 1995, the number of seriously overweight children and adolescents has more than doubled in the past decade. The study—which examined a national sample of 2,920 young people from 1988 to 1991—found that 4.7 million American youths aged six through seventeen are severely overweight.

To put it simply, kids today are fatter and less fit than ever before. There are many factors contributing to this disturbing trend:

1. Gym class is no longer a mandatory part of every American school's curriculum.
2. There are fewer safe and clean playgrounds and recreation facilities then when I was a kid.
3. Organized sports aren't affordable for all families.
4. The rise in sedentary activities—playing video games, watching television, and spending hours in front of a computer.
5. Bad eating habits (what you'd call junk food junkies).

The result is a generation of unhealthy—and obese—children. (This is not to say that all kids should be skinny, of course. But being significantly overweight is definitely not healthy, and it sets kids up for more serious health risks later in life.)

The 1996 Surgeon General's Report on Physical Activity and Health found that 50 percent of American kids do not engage in physical activity appropriate to long-term health promotion, and about fifteen percent aren't active at all. Much of this is due to the fact that adults aren't setting good examples for kids. In short, we are becoming a nation of unhealthy adults producing unhealthy children. We all know that the behaviors children see at home are the ones they most often adopt for themselves. Let's not just tell kids about good nutrition and being active, let's show them. Make it a family affair. Helping kids develop good eating and fitness habits at an early age is the best thing we can do to ensure that our children—and their children—grow up healthy and strong.

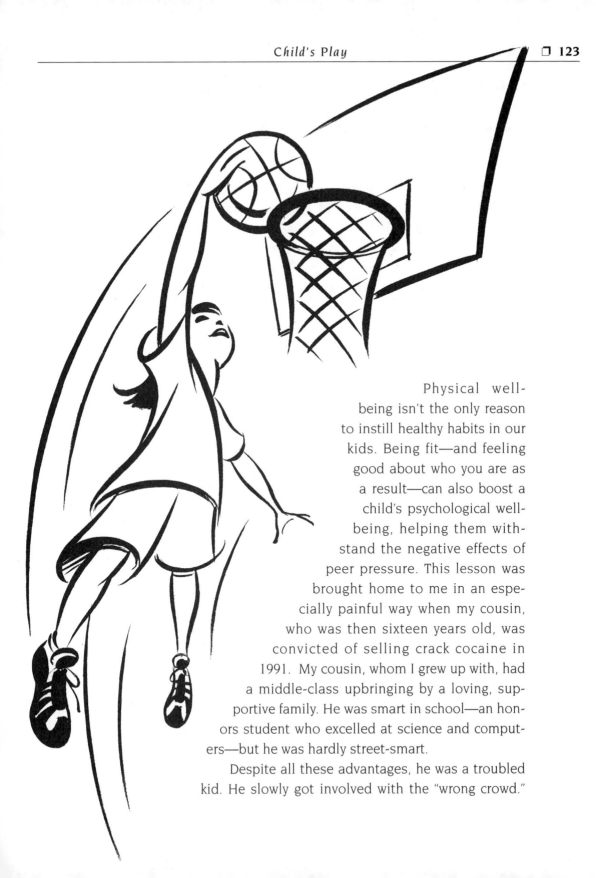

Physical well-being isn't the only reason to instill healthy habits in our kids. Being fit—and feeling good about who you are as a result—can also boost a child's psychological well-being, helping them withstand the negative effects of peer pressure. This lesson was brought home to me in an especially painful way when my cousin, who was then sixteen years old, was convicted of selling crack cocaine in 1991. My cousin, whom I grew up with, had a middle-class upbringing by a loving, supportive family. He was smart in school—an honors student who excelled at science and computers—but he was hardly street-smart.

Despite all these advantages, he was a troubled kid. He slowly got involved with the "wrong crowd."

When some friends challenged him to prove he was cool by experimenting with—and eventually selling—drugs, my cousin didn't have the inner strength to just walk away. He was arrested and spent some time in prison before going into a rehab facility. Despite receiving help to get his life back on track, my cousin ended up choosing life in the fast lane. When I think of all the possibilities that were open to this bright, young kid—and the fact that he's chosen to throw his future away by using and selling drugs—it really breaks my heart.

Instead of sitting on the sidelines doing nothing, I took action. My cousin's experience inspired me to start my StayFit Kids Program, which aims to help kids excel not just on the playing field, but also in life. I began hosting free lectures, demonstrations, and fitness clinics for kids around the world. My goal is to make a difference in children's lives, and to keep kids like my cousin from losing their way. (You know, it's the whole "a strong body = a strong mind" connection.)

Let's focus on building kids up and not letting them down. To help kids succeed, we must teach them how to take control of their lives and how to reach their fullest potential. Repairing the damage done to our youth's vitality and self-worth will not be an easy job. But I've discovered, through my own efforts to promote positive lifestyles through fitness, that this task is not insurmountable.

Another problem, one that is more common—and far more unhealthy—than eating poorly and being sedentary, is having a bad self-image. This issue affects almost everyone living in America today, regardless of age. Much of our self-image is derived from our feelings about our bodies—and most of us aren't too happy with the way we look. This sense of physical dissatisfaction is especially prevalent among women, who are expected to look a certain way in order to be considered attractive or desirable by today's standards (read: young and thin) .

An unrealistic desire for physical perfection is beginning to have a dangerous effect on even the youngest members of our society. A recent study by the University of Arizona found that more than half of the teenage girls polled had tried to lose weight within the past year, and that 90 percent of the white teens and 30 percent of the black teens polled were dissatisfied with their weight or shape. Even more disturbing is the American Dietetic Association's announcement that children as young as six and seven are already concerned with their body image and are afraid of gaining weight. By age nine, four out of five girls have already been on a self-imposed diet to lose weight. This is a serious issue, especially considering that only one out of four of these children is actually overweight. The rest, according to the ADA, suffer from a distorted body image. It's time we took the focus off of weight and put it back where it belongs—on good health. The bottom line is this: being underweight is just as unhealthy as being overweight.

This focus on outward appearance—whether it begins in childhood or later in life—affects most of us at one time or another. The effect is almost always detrimental to our overall well-being. Regardless of your size or shape or other people's perceptions, you have to love yourself. I really do believe that when you nurture from within, that energy transcends out. Even people who look fit and are physically healthy can be plagued with a negative self-image. While looks sometimes are deceiving, good health radiates naturally—and this holds true whether you're eight or eighty-eight.

What Can You Do to Help?

At Home

First let's take care of business. When you're at home with your kids, turn off the TV and get with the program. The number one thing you can do to ensure that your children are physically active is to be active yourself. It's a lot easier for kids to watch television or play a video game than it is for them to get up, go outside, and play. (In fact, according to a Texas Instruments study, the average third grader watches 1,170 hours of TV each year—that's roughly 23 hours each week—and spends only 900 hours a year in school.) There are many activities competing for a child's time and attention. To motivate kids to be active, you have to be active yourself and set an example. If you talk the talk, you gotta walk the walk. (And you are walking, right?) As with other early childhood behaviors, children will "follow the leader." Children will develop healthy habits when the activities are reinforced by parents who not only advocate—but also participate in—sports and fitness with their kids. In fact, in a 1995 Gallup poll, entitled "What Kid's Think," 59 percent of children who were active responded that it was their family who encouraged them to get involved in sports, recreational activities, or exercise.

Of course, I've also seen many folks who spend a lot of time and money getting in shape and looking good, yet they have children who are overweight. "Oh, my kid will outgrow that," they tell me. I'm telling you now that they *won't*. Unless you invest in their health, like you have in your own, they'll just grow up to be fat adults who don't have enough energy to reach for the brass ring. For the sake of yourself and your kids, it's important to make regular physical activity and healthy eating an important part of your family's lifestyle. It's a family thing!

The next time you tell your kids to "go outside and play," why not go out with them? Take your kids biking, swimming, in-line skating, or go out and shoot some hoops with them. Plan weekends and vacations with your kids where everyone gets to choose activities that the entire family will enjoy. Making choices, acting on them, and learning through the consequences of one's actions are ongoing processes that begin in early childhood and continue for a lifetime.

Children use play to figure out how their world works and how they fit into that world. Through play, children gain a sense of competence and control over their lives. They learn to interact with others and resolve conflicts, develop their imaginations, and foster creativity. Also, look into signing up your kids to play in organized sports, which is a means of improving socialization and developing discipline and teamwork skills. Play is a dynamic process by which children learn to learn. As with anything else, children can develop good fitness habits that they'll carry into adulthood.

It's important to remember that kids will mimic your eating habits, as well. If they see you sitting in front of the boob tube every afternoon scarfing down a big ol' bag of chips, they'll want some, too. Why wouldn't they? If, on the other hand, you make a point of eating well by following the USDA Food Guide Pyramid (outlined in the next chapter), your child is more likely to do the same. Remember, the only difference is that children need to get *at least* the minimum number of servings from each food group *every* day to ensure proper growth. Youngsters will copy many of your habits, likes and dislikes. When it comes to making wise food choices, your actions speak louder than words. Practice what you preach, and your actions will make *you* healthier, too!

Oh, by the way, did I mention it may be a *lit-tle* challenging to lure them away from watching TV or talking on the phone? Fear not, I have a fail-proof solution: if you appeal to their sense of fun and adventure, you're well on your way. The main thing to remember here is: it has to be fun. I'm a big kid at heart, and in addition to working hard, I play hard. Playing is a great form of physical activity. It helps rejuvenate us, both physically and emotionally, after long work weeks. It's the perfect way to provide the three R's that are necessary for relieving stress: rest, relaxation, and recreation. Look for activities that are simple, fun, and amusing. Here are a few examples of fun activities that you and your family can do together:

Fitness scavenger hunt. Put a new twist on an old idea by having your kids perform some problem-solving games that require physical activity, teamwork, and decision-making skills.

Birthday fitness party. Hold a wacky backyard fitness carnival with a basketball shoot, baseball or football toss, three-legged, sack, and wheelbarrow races. Use your imagination to help build your child's level of skill-related fitness.

Imitate an animal contest (for younger kids). Some of the movements that you can do involve galloping like a horse, walking "tall" on your toes like a giraffe, and hopping like a frog. Movements like these help develop the motor skills required for good physical development, and they also involve a lot of creativity.

Obstacle course. Crawling through Hula Hoops, jumping over ropes, walking on an imaginary balance beam, and tumbling are all useful skills for building confidence and risk-taking behavior.

If you're looking for more structured activities, here are some other examples of fun-filled family adventures:

- ◆ Go camping
- ◆ Go on a nature trail hike
- ◆ Go canoeing or ride a paddle boat
- ◆ Go horseback riding
- ◆ Go on a ski trip
- ◆ Go to an amusement park
- ◆ The key word here is *Go!*

Use your imagination and get your whole family involved in making physical activity a lifetime pursuit. Remember, you're only as old as you think and feel. Miss D's Rx for the fountain of youth? Go out and play!

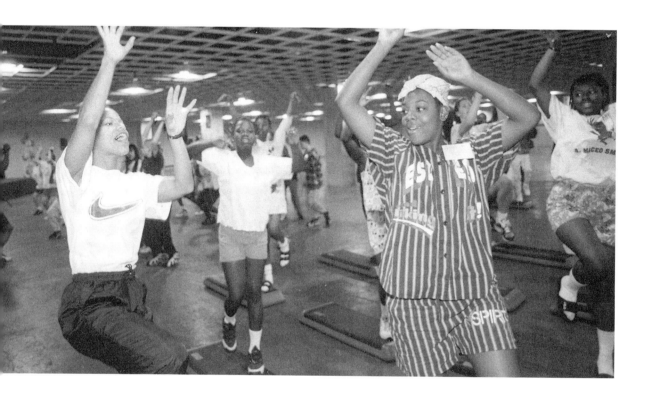

Keeping Kids Healthy

Adults aren't the only ones who need to work physical activity into their daily lives. Kids have to make an effort to be more active, too. Here are some cool exercises for your children to try:

H$_2$0 Curl

1. Hold one water bottle in each hand, palms facing forward. Sit on the edge of a chair with your feet flat on the floor and your arms extended down at your sides.

2. Lift the water bottles toward your shoulders, keeping your elbows at your side, then lower back down. Breathe out as you lift the bottles up and breathe in as you lower them back down. Repeat twelve times. This exercise strengthens the bicep muscles in your upper arm.

The Dip

1. The next time you get restless while studying at your desk, just dip it! Sit on the edge of your seat with your hands resting flat on the front of the chair, palms down and fingers facing forward. Your knees should be bent and your feet should be flat on the floor.

2. Hold on to the chair and lift your buttocks off the seat. Bend your elbows and lower your tailbone down toward the floor until you're a few inches off the ground. Then push yourself back up by staightening out your arms. Repeat twelve times without resting between dips. Breathe out as you push up and breathe in as you dip down. This exercise works the back part of your upper arm (triceps).

Squat and Sit

1. Do this exercise before you sit down at your desk or at the dinner table. Stand straight in front of a chair with your feet placed shoulder-width apart.

2. Pretend that you're going to sit down, but stop just before your buttocks touch the seat. Keep your torso straight, and stand up straight again. Breathe in as you squat down, and exhale as you stand up. Repeat twelve times. This exercise strengthens the quadricep muscle in the front part of your thigh, the hamstring muscle in the back of your thigh, and your gluteus maximus (butt) muscle.

Crunch Time

1. The next time you're watching your favorite TV show, do some crunches during the commercial break. (And you know I'm not talking about eating some Cap'n Crunch, so don't even try to

play that with Miss Donna.) Lie on your back on the floor. Your knees should be bent, your feet flat, and your hands crossed over your chest.

2. Raise your head and shoulder blades off the floor while tightening your stomach muscles. Breathe out when you lift up and breathe in when you lie back. Repeat twelve times. Keep your lower back on the floor at all times, and don't arch it. This exercise strengthens your stomach muscles and will make your abs look totally awesome.

Push It

1. Aside from doing crunches during commercials, see how many push-ups you can do during the break. Start by kneeling on the floor with your ankles crossed and your hands flat on the floor at shoulder height. Keep your abs tight, your back straight, and your head in line with your shoulders.

2. Bend your arms at the elbow and lower your chest until your torso is almost touching the floor. Straighten your arms out, then repeat again. Breathe out when you straighten your arms and breathe in when you bend them. This exercise strengthens your chest (pectoral), shoulder (deltoid), and upper arm (tricep) muscles. (If bent-knee push-ups are too easy, you can do "military" push-ups by resting on your hands and your feet.) Who said you can't do two things at once? Exercising while you watch TV is fun and convenient.

Remote Control Stretch

1. To ward off any upper back tightness, sit on the couch with the remote in your left hand.

2. Stretch your arm to the far-left corner of the room. Your body should still be facing the television (no twisting, puh-leeze!). Hold for several seconds, then lower your arm.

3. Switch the remote to your right hand, and repeat with your right arm.

Bedspread Stretch

1. Don't throw a fit the next time Mom nags you to make your bed. Instead, use it to stretch out your leg muscles. Place your left foot on top of the pile of dirty clothes on your bed, keeping your standing leg slightly bent.

2. Bend forward at the hip and reach for your toes—but don't bounce. You should feel the stretch in the hamstring muscles in the back of your thigh. Hold for several seconds, then switch to the other leg and repeat.

Note: When you do all of the above exercises, do them slowly, in a controlled manner. Don't jerk it, don't bounce it. Keep it smooth.

In School

During the mid-1980s, I was hired by a school's PTA to set up a weekly fitness program that combined traditional gym class activities with aerobics and calisthenics. We played volleyball and kickball; I got mini-trampolines, and those kids jumped for joy. After each class, I'd assign homework designed to teach them how the human body works. The youngest children, for instance, might be asked to go home and find Mom's and Dad's resting heart rates. The older kids might be asked to draw a strong, healthy body and label all the parts. The goal of that program was to provide a fun-filled learning environment that promoted positive health habits and good attitudes that the kids would carry throughout life.

I worked to further that goal by volunteering as a spokesperson for Nike's P.L.A.Y. (Participate in the Lives of America's Youth) program, which is designed to keep recreation alive for kids by creating opportunities for them to learn to be fit and healthy. I also helped put together the American Council on Exercise's Energy 2 Burn program, which has been implemented in schools across the country. Energy 2 Burn is a new fitness program that uses classroom activity and a high-energy video to get kids off the couch and show them how to make exercise a part of their daily routine. It teaches them to think of exercise as fun, not a daily chore.

In addition to teaching public and private school students, I also volunteered to work with disadvantaged teenagers at a special school in Washington, D.C. It was a "last chance" school for kids who had been released from detention centers or kicked out of public schools. Some were homeless and some came from abusive backgrounds—talk about a challenging situation. These kids had incredible problems, but many of them just didn't want to be (or didn't think that they deserved to be) helped. I designed my StayFit Kids program to increase the kids' self-esteem by helping them learn to love and respect themselves. Only by educating young minds and instilling in them a sincere passion for a healthy, balanced, and positive lifestyle can we begin to remedy the dangers of an unhealthy, unstable childhood.

StayFit Kids also stresses the importance of staying in school and getting a good education. An education is the passport to a brighter future. (To all you naysayers, I am practicing what I preach. I recently went back to school to complete my undergraduate degree. Although I've had a pretty successful career, I made a commitment to finish what I started. At this moment, I'm feeling mighty good because my diploma is glowing from its place of honor on my office wall.)

My first day at this school was really scary. These kids had total disregard for everyone and everything. I videotaped our first session together, and then I played it for them at the next class. I said, "Look at your behavior. The camera doesn't lie." The tape showed them mouthing off and hitting each other; one girl even called me a bitch. It really hurt me to see kids who just totally disrespected me, as well as themselves. After a while the whole room became quiet. I said, "You know, in order for me to help you, you've got to want to help yourselves. If I were to send this videotape out, is this the way that you would want yourself represented?"

The answer, of course, was no. The kids agreed to to work with me. I established rules and guidelines for them to follow, and told them they could either get with the program or miss out on the fun. In the beginning, every day presented another problem or challenge—worrying about someone stealing my car, finding one of my female students having sex on school grounds. But as we continued to work together, their behavior—and sense of self-worth—slowly started to improve. I began by talking with them about different problems they faced: pregnancy, death, drugs, and any problems they were having in school or with their parents. We always followed each rap session with a workout.

I've spoken with mayors and city councilmen across the country, and they're always talking about installing more metal detectors and positioning more police officers in schools. Forget that crap. Start with their heads, and their hearts and bodies will follow. I don't care how many cops and metal detectors you have, if we want kids to put down the knives and guns, we have to help them to feel good about who they are and what they can become. That sense of self-worth begins on the *inside*.

I understand that certain schools need security in order to protect the students and faculty, but let's focus on the long-term solution. What I learned from working at this school (and others) is that what kids need more than anything else is to be loved and cared for. They need to have someone there to encourage them—to help them believe in themselves and in their potential to achieve. *You could be that someone.* It's only when kids believe that they're worth something that they'll begin to take care of their minds and bodies. Working with kids who are less fortunate than I am has made me very thankful for what I have. When some problem arises in my life, I often find myself thinking, "Is this situation really worth stressing over? I mean, the kid you were with yesterday told you his family couldn't afford dinner last night." It really puts things in perspective.

In the Community

In addition to promoting physical education within the school system, parents can also have an impact on the community at large. Spearhead efforts to facilitate and support organized sports and recreational activities geared toward the younger generation. Unfortunately, government budget cuts have forced many once-thriving community centers to close their doors, and the rise in violent and drug-related crimes have turned many parks and recreational areas into dangerous war zones. But many national organizations are stepping in to help parents help their children find a safe place to play. Contact your mayors, congressman, and senators, and get them involved in improving our kids' health and well-being.

Through my travels, I've helped organize many programs geared toward helping kids around the world. In Bogotá, Colombia, I worked with local fitness pros to help improve the welfare of homeless kids. We lead Sunday fitness festivals in the park—where many of these kids, unfortunately, lived on their own. Folks from all walks of life were invited to stop by and participate in the sessions. After leading a fitness class and teaching the virtues of a healthy lifestyle and the importance of reaching out to those less fortunate, my colleagues and I handed out trash bags and encouraged everyone to pitch in and help clean up the park. The program has had a very positive impact on the community and has inspired a mentoring program, a homeless shelter for kids, and has taught people to be more responsible for the environment. People helping people is what we need a little bit more of today.

We have a responsibility to help our children. Instead of waiting to take action, be a part of the solution. There are plenty of things you can do to help. Volunteer at your local Boys & Girls Club, or join a mentor program, such as Big Brothers/Big Sisters of America, which pairs girls and boys with women and men who act as role models and friends. You could also volunteer to work with kids at a school or community center in your neighborhood. Contact your local parks department and offer to conduct programs, or help with activities they've already planned. Malls frequently sponsor special events or demonstrations; design a youth-activity plan and discuss it with the mall manager. And yes, you can always donate money to a local or national children's program, such as mine. Together, we can make a difference by helping to improve the quality of young people's lives. As Franklin D. Roosevelt once said, "We cannot always build the future for our youth, but we can build our youth for the future."

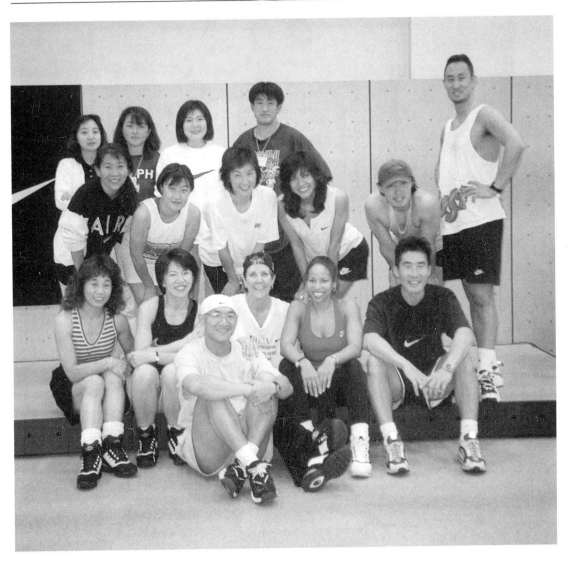

Doing good work with my colleagues in Tokyo.

8

Nutrition 101

Now that we've covered the basics of a well-rounded fitness routine, you probably think that you know all there is to know about getting and staying healthy, right? *Wrong.* Exercise is only half of the story. Eating well is equally important for maintaining good health.

Now, I'm sure that many of you rolled your eyes at the phrase "eating well." I can almost hear the collective moan. "Oh, great," you're thinking, "now comes the part where she tells us that we have to give up red meat and ice cream." While that "all or nothing" thinking may be popular with trendy diet doctors, it's not a theory to which I subscribe.

You'll never catch me telling people that they have to subsist on rabbit food (although I do love my veggies), or that they should put themselves on a starvation diet in order to lose twenty pounds in a month. The reason? Extreme, restrictive diets don't work. Sure, it's great to increase your veggie intake, but if that's *all* you eat, you'll deprive yourself of other nutrients that are equally important. (Vegetarians, for instance, always have to make sure that they get enough nutrients—especially protein.) Likewise, if you're anything like me, and you tell yourself that you can never ever eat a thick, juicy steak again, then eating a thick, juicy steak is *all* you'll be thinking about. In my mind, there are *no can'ts*—not when it comes to fitness, and not when it comes to food. But before you order that large pizza with extra cheese and pepperoni, read on.

Food is fuel. Your body can't function without fuel now, can it? That would be like trying to run your car on an empty tank of gas—it ain't gonna work.

The Seven Types of Nutrients

There are seven types of nutrients that are necessary to maintain good health: carbohydrates, protein, fiber, fats, minerals, vitamins, and water. To help you understand the importance of these nutrients, you first have to understand just how your body uses them.

Carbohydrates

Carbohydrates are one of the main sources of fuel for your muscles. Because your body stores only small amounts of this nutrient, you must replenish your supply by eating plenty of carbodyhdrate-containing foods. Breads, grains, cereals, pastas, vegetables, and legumes (beans) are good sources of *complex* carbohydrates. Complex carbs are low in calories and fat, and high in fiber. Your digestive system breaks down the carbohydrates you eat into sugar, and it's this sugar that gives your body the energy it needs to function. The sugar found in complex carbs is absorbed into your bloodstream slowly, which means that your energy level is boosted for quite a while—and you feel full longer, to boot.

The sugar found in *simple* carbohydrates, on the other hand, is absorbed into your bloodstream lickety-split. Your blood sugar level skyrockets then nosedives (which leaves you feeling hungry and cranky). Simple carbs occur naturally in fruits and can also be found in table sugar and processed foods such as soft drinks and candy bars. Processed sweet treats may taste good doing down, but they'll leave you feeling testy and tired in the long run.

Protein

We need protein for a number of reasons: to repair and build body tissues; to produce enzymes, hormones, and other substances the body uses; to regulate body processes such as water balance; to transport nutrients; and to make the muscles contract. Most athletes need slightly more protein than nonathletes (three to four servings per day, as opposed to two to three servings for moderately active folks). Good sources of protein are lean meats, poultry, fish, low-fat cheese, dairy products (low-fat or nonfat varieties are the best choices), legumes, tofu, and eggs. And keep in mind that while there has been a lot of attention given to the newly popular low carb/high protein diets, there is no scientific proof to back up claims that these diets are any healthier or more effective than the food recommendations made by the United States Department of Agriculture (USDA).

Fiber

Fiber is the nondigestible or partially digestible material found in plant cells, and it comes from three specific food groups: fruits, vegetables, and whole grain breads and cereals. As you're probably aware, fiber helps keep you regular. Since it's naturally low fat and very filling, it doesn't take much to make you feel full. Fiber is also thought to prevent heart disease and colon cancer by moving harmful waste out of our systems quickly.

A word of caution: when it comes to fiber, a little goes a long way. If you're not currently eating a high-fiber diet, it's best to increase your intake gradually (or you may find yourself spending a lot of extra time in the bathroom).

Fat

Unless you've been living under a rock without access to a newspaper or a television for the past ten years, you've undoubtedly heard about any number of scientific studies that have shown how bad a high-fat diet is for the human body. While there is no doubt that excessive fat intake is unhealthy—it can increase the risk of heart disease, obesity, and other health problems—many people mistakenly believe that they need to cut fat out of their diets entirely to be healthy. This is definitely untrue and downright *un*healthy.

Fat is an essential nutrient. Our bodies need it in order to function properly. In addition to providing essential fatty acids, which the body cannot manufacture, fat carries fat-soluble vitamins (A, D, E, and K) needed for proper growth and development. Fats act as an insulator to maintain body temperature, aid in digestion, and provide the greatest energy output per gram of any food source. (They also contribute important taste and texture qualities that make eating so enjoyable.)

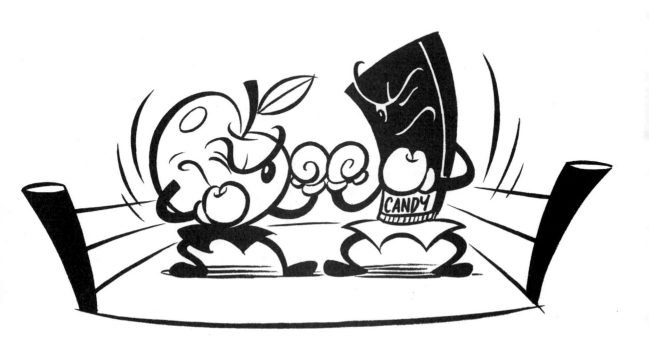

A Note On Cholesterol

While fats are found in both animal and vegetable sources, cholesterol is found *only* in animal products such as eggs, meat, poultry, fish, dairy products, butter, and lard. Margarine and cooking oil *never* contain cholesterol. It should be noted, however, that the cholesterol in food is not a major cause of high blood cholesterol for most individuals. Unfortunately, the same cannot be said of saturated fat. Saturated fat tends to raise blood cholesterol levels, so reducing saturated fat intake is extremely important. Polyunsaturated fats, on the other hand, have been proven to reduce blood cholesterol levels, and monounsaturated fats may indirectly lower blood cholesterol if they are used to replace saturated fat in the diet.

To ensure good health, your blood cholesterol levels should be under 200 milligrams per deciliter. A total cholesterol level between 200 and 239 milligrams per deciliter is considered borderline high, and a level of 240 and above is considered dangerously high. People with high blood cholesterol are twice as likely to develop coronary heart disease as are people in the optimal range.

Briefly, the different types of fats break down as follows:

Saturated. Most are solid at room temperature. Saturated fats cause the blood cholesterol levels to rise (and elevated cholesterol levels are the primary cause of heart disease). Common saturated fats include animal fats, palm oil, palm kernel oil, and coconut oil.

Unsaturated. Most are liquid at room temperature. Unsaturated fats do not elevate blood cholesterol level, but they can contribute to obesity if not eaten in moderation. Examples of unsaturated fats are:

    Monounsaturated — olive oil, peanut oil, canola oil
    Polyunsaturated — corn oil, safflower oil, soybean oil, cottonseed
        oil, sunflower oil, and sesame oil

Health experts recommend that Americans consume 30 percent or less of their total daily calories from fat, with 10 percent or less of those calories coming from saturated fat. The 30 percent refers to total fat intake over the course of the day, not to individual foods or meals. The goal is to consume a moderate amount of fat, not to have a totally fat-free diet. (In fact, last year, the American Heart Association began recommending that people consume a *mininimum* amount of 15 percent fat daily.) Use the Nutrition Facts panel on food labels to help determine how much fat is in the foods you eat. Remember, it's the total fat intake over time that's important—not the amount of fat in one particular food. A food that is high in fat can be part of a healthy diet as long as it's balanced with other lower-fat food choices.

A Note on Fat-Free Foods

In the past few years, there seems to have been a sudden surge in the number of low-fat and fat-free foods on the market. It's important to remember, however, that fat-free does not mean calorie-free. (Translation: just because it's low-fat doesn't mean you should devour the entire box in one sitting.) I know all too well the temptation of eating an entire box of Snackwell's low-fat miniature chocolate chip cookies. My friends always say I should have stock in the company.

Vitamins and Minerals

Ideally, you should be getting all of your vitamins and minerals directly from the source (meaning from the foods you eat). As we all know, that isn't always possible. Between juggling the demands of our professional and personal lives, many of us often don't even have time to eat, let alone eat right! If you want to be sure that you're getting all the nutrients your body needs to function properly, you may want to take a daily multivitamin. I've been taking multivitamins every morning since I was a kid. I like knowing that no matter how hectic my schedule gets, I've already given my body the vitamins it needs to get the job done.

U.S. Recommended Daily Allowance (RDA) for Vitamins and Minerals

VITAMIN	RDA WOMEN	RDA MEN
A (beta carotene)	800 IU	1000 IU
B_1 (thiamine)	1.1 mg	1.5 mg
B_2 (riboflavin)	1.3 mg	1.7 mg
B_6 (pyridoxine)	1.6 mg	2.0 mg
B_{12}	2.0 mg	2.0 mg
C (ascorbic acid)	60 mg	60 mg
D	5 IU	5 IU
E	8 mg	10 mg
Folic acid	180 IU	200 IU
K	64 IU	80 IU
Niacin	15 mg	19 mg

MINERALS		
Calcium	800 mg	800 mg
Chromium	RDA not established	RDA n/a
Copper	RDA not established	RDA n/a
Iodine	150 IU	150 IU
Iron	15 mg	10 mg
Magnesium	280 mg	350 mg
Phosphorus	800 mg	800 mg
Potassium	RDA not established	RDA n/a
Selenium	55 IU	70 IU
Zinc	12 mg	15 mg

Good Natural Food Sources of Vitamins and Minerals

VITAMIN	FUNCTIONS	SOURCES
A (retinol)	Helps maintain eyes, skin, linings of the nose, mouth, digestive, and urinary tracts.	Liver, whole milk, butter, cheese, fortified margarine, carrots, spinach
Thiamin (B_1)	Helps convert carbohydrates into energy.	Yeast, rice, whole grain breads and cereals, liver, pork, poultry, eggs, fish, fruits and vegetables
Riboflavin (B_2)	Helps energy release; helps maintain skin, mucuous membranes, and nervous structures.	Dairy products, liver, yeast, fruits, whole grain breads and cereals, vegetables, lean meats, poultry
Niacin (B_3)	Helps convert carbohydrates, fats, and protein into energy; essential for growth; aids synthesis of hormones.	Liver, chicken, turkey, halibut, tuna, milk, eggs, grains, fruits and vegetables, enriched breads and cereals
B_6 (pyridoxine, pyridoxamine	Aids in more than 60 enzyme reactions.	Milk, liver, lean meats, whole grain breads and cereals, vegetables
Folic acid	Aids blood-cell production; helps maintain nervous system.	Liver, many vegetables
Biotin	Aids in intermediary metabolism of carboyhdrates, fats and protein.	Widely distributed in foods
Pantothenic acid	Aids in metabolism of carbohydrates, fats, and protein.	Eggs, liver, kidneys, peanuts, whole grains, most vegetables, fish
B_{12}	Helps synthesize red and white bood cells; aids many metabolic reactions.	Liver, meat, eggs, milk
C (ascorbic acid)	Helps maintain and repair connective tissue, bones, teeth, cartilage; promotes healing.	Broccoli, brussels sprouts, citrus fruits and vegetables

VITAMIN	FUNCTIONS	SOURCES
D (cholecalciferol)	Helps regulate calcium and phosphorus metabolism; essential for bones and teeth.	Fortified milk, fish-liver oils; sunlight on skin produces vitamin D
E (tocopherol)	Protects and maintains cellular membranes.	Vegetable oils, whole grains, leafy vegetables
K	Used in synthesis of prothrombin (essential for blood clotting).	Green leafy vegetables, soybeans, beef liver, widespread in foods
Calcium	Builds and maintains strong bones, prevents osteoporosis.	Dairy products, leafy green vegetables, broccoli, dried fruit
Chromium	Helps break down carbs so your body can use them as an energy source.	Meat, clams, cheese, nuts, brewer's yeast
Copper	Boosts your immune system and regulates cholesterol levels.	Shellfish, whole grains, organ meats, fruits, fish, vegetables, nuts, lean meats, legumes
Iodine	Helps regulate your metabolism.	Iodized salt, seafood, dairy, meats seaweed
Iron	Keeps blood healthy and boosts immunity.	Organ meats, red meat, shellfish, egg yolks, dried fruits, leafy green vegetables, enriched cereals, poultry
Magnesium	Protects against heart disease and kidney stones.	Whole grains, nuts, legumes, dark green leafy vegetables, seafood, chocolate
Phosphorus	Builds strong bones and teeth, helps transmit nerve impulses.	Meat, fish, dairy, egg yolks, nuts, poultry, legumes, whole grains
Potassium	Lowers blood pressure.	Lean meat, dairy, nuts, fresh fruits, and vegetables, legumes
Selenium	Acts as an antioxidant.	Seafood, lean meats, organ meat, dairy
Zinc	Maintains your sense of taste.	Lobster, oysters, crab, extra-lean beef, dark turkey meat

Diet and Disease Prevention

I've already told you which foods contain what vitamins and how they work to keep the body healthy. Here's a brief look at how vitamins aid in disease prevention.

Vitamin	Established Benefit	Possible Benefit
A (beta carotene)	Prevents night blindness and xerophthalmia (a common cause of blindness among children in poor countries).	May reduce the risk of breast, lung, colon, prostate and cervical cancer, heart disease and stroke; may retard macular degeneration (a common cause of blindness in the elderly).
B₆	Helps prevent anemia, skin lesions, nerve damage.	May protect against neural-tube defects in fetuses.
B₁₂	Helps prevent pernicious anemia.	May protect against heart disease and nerve damage. Possibly prevents neural-tube defects in fetuses during the first six weeks of pregnancy.
C	Prevents scurvy, loose teeth; fights hemorrhage.	May help reduce the risk of cancer and heart disease; retards macular degeneration in the eyes of the elderly.
D	Prevents rickets (bone malformation).	May help prevent osteoporosis and kidney disease.
E	Helps prevent retrolental fibroplasia (an eye disorder in premature infants), anemia.	May reduce risk of angina and heart attack; may slow macular degeneration; may prevent spinal-cord damage in patients with cystic fibrosis.
Folic acid	Helps protect against cervical dysplasia (precancerous changes in cells of the uterine cervix).	May help protect against heart disease, nerve damage, neural tube defects.
K	Helps prevent hemorrhage.	Possible role in cancer prevention.
Niacin	Prevents pellagra (a disease of the central nervous system).	Possible cancer inhibitor.

If you're not meeting your daily nutritional requirements and are not able to get them through dietary measures alone, you should definitely think about taking supplements. Vitamin supplements are especially important if you suffer from anemia, or if you don't get enough calcium in your diet. Just be careful not to overdo it, and always check with your doctor before taking supplements.

Taking megadoses of some vitamins can actually do more harm than good. Too high a dose of one vitamin can inhibit the absorption of another, and certain vitamins, if consumed in excessive amounts, can have undesirable side effects, such as fatigue, diarrhea, and hair loss. Others may cause more serious side effects such as kidney stones, liver or neurological damage, birth defects, or even death. To be on the safe side, stick with a basic multivitamin (iron- or calcium-enriched if necessary) that gives you no more than 100 percent of the Recommended Daily Allowance.

Don't Forget Water!

In addition to fueling your body with the nutrients it needs to run smoothly, you also need to make sure you drink enough liquids—especially water. Water is a vital ingredient in maintaining good health. It regulates body temperature, carries nutrients and oxygen to cells, and removes wastes. It also cushions joints and protects organs and tissues. Everyone should drink at least eight eight-ounce (one cup) glasses of water each and every day (and you need to drink an additional one to three cups per hour if you're working out).

People who are exposed to extreme climates—either hot or cold—also need more water because the body has to work harder to maintain a normal temperature in those conditions. Likewise, prolonged exposure to heated or recirculated air creates a drying effect that draws extra fluid out of the skin, which needs to replenished more frequently. Extra fluid is needed if you are pregnant or breast-feeding—or if you eat a high-fiber diet (extra water is needed to process the additional roughage and to prevent constipation).

Healthy Eating Made Easy

Instead of fad diets and doomed-to-fail gizmos (what's in all those diet pills, anyway!??), I recommend adopting healthier eating habits based on the USDA's Food Guide Pyramid. The Food Guide Pyramid is a practical tool that's designed to help you make food choices that are in keeping with government-sanctioned dietary guidelines for Americans. According to the USDA, healthy eating is dependent on *balance, variety,* and *moderation.*

Balance refers to incorporating all the major food groups into your daily diet. Since the recommended servings are different for every food group, you need to make sure you're eating the proper number of servings from each one.

Variety refers to choosing a selection of foods from each of the major food groups, while minimizing the calories from fats, oils, and sweets.

Moderation refers to choosing a diet low in fat, cholesterol, sugar, sodium, and alcohol—food components that have been linked to chronic disease. Moderation, as the word implies, also means eating moderate portion sizes. The amount you should eat depends upon your individual caloric needs, as well as your activity level (the more calories you burn being active, the more you need to eat, in order to maintain your weight and energy level).

Here's how the different food groups stack-up, calorically:

Source of Calories	Calories per Gram
Fat	9
Carbohydrate	4
Protein	4

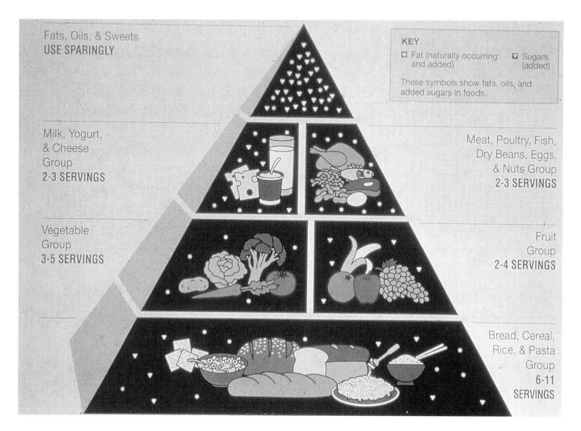

Source: U.S. Department of Agriculture/U.S. Department of Health and Human Services

To make the most of the Food Guide Pyramid, you need to know what counts as a serving.

FOOD GROUP	SERVING SIZE
Grains	1 slice bread; $1/2$ bagel, hamburger bun, or English muffin; 1 tortilla, dinner roll or small muffin; 1 oz. dry cereal; $1/2$ cup cooked cereal, rice, or pasta; 5 to 6 small crackers
Vegetable	1 cup raw, leafy vegetables; $1/2$ cup cooked or chopped raw vegetables; $3/4$ cup vegetable juice; 1 medium potato
Fruit	1 medium piece of fruit; $1/2$ cup mixed or canned fruit; $1/2$ grapefruit; $1/4$ cantaloupe; $1/4$ cup raisins or dry fruit; $1/4$ cup fruit juice
Milk	1 cup milk or yogurt; $1^{1}/2$ ounces natural cheese or 2 ounces processed cheese; $1/2$ cup cottage cheese; $1/2$ cup ice cream, ice milk, or frozen yogurt
Meat	2 to 3 ounces cooked lean meat, poultry, or fish. Other foods that count as 1 ounce meat: $1/2$ cup cooked dry beans, 1 egg, 2 table spoons peanut butter, $1/3$ cup nuts

There are many factors that determine your weight, including your sex, height, age, and genetic composition. As you've already learned, excess body fat increases the risk of high blood pressure, heart disease, stroke, diabetes, some types of cancer, and other illnesses (a topic I cover in detail in chapter 10). But being too thin isn't any better; it can increase the risk of osteoporosis, menstrual irregularities, and other health problems. Likewise, "yo-yo" dieting (losing and regaining weight over and over again) wreaks havoc with your metabolism and can actually make you fatter than if you'd never dieted at all ("The horror! The horror!"). So what's the real secret to maintaining a steady, healthy weight? Again and again and again, it's all about *moderation*.

If your favorite foods are high in fat, salt, or sugar, don't try to eliminate them from your diet. Moderate *how much* of these foods you eat, and *how often* you eat them. If, like me, you love pizza, you don't have to give it up. Just eat it less often and try to balance it with other foods. Sometimes when I'm eating at a restaurant and I indulge in pizza or key lime pie, I get dirty looks from women who are probably thinking, "She's one of those people who can eat anything she wants and never gain a pound!" The same thing happens when I shop for clothes. I've had sales assistants literally roll their eyes when I ask for my size. The truth is, I *cannot* and *do not* eat anything I want. But I do treat myself to the foods I love every once in a while, and you should too. (As for my body, it's the product of good genes and *lots* of hard work.)

Smart Snacks

It's important to eat regular meals. *Regular* used to refer to three distinct meals—breakfast, lunch, and dinner—but these days, it's really a matter of personal preference. Some folks prefer eating three "squares" a day, while others like to "graze" (eat small servings of different types of food five or six times a day). Many people find that grazing keeps their energy level on an even keel throughout the day and helps counteract that midafternoon slump.

Whatever your preference, don't skip meals. Your body uses up the carbohydrate stores in your liver (which help maintain a normal blood sugar level) in four to six hours, and you need food to replace them. Keeping healthy snacks—such as fruit, pretzels, or low-fat yogurt—on hand will help prevent a junk food binge, and they'll definitely put some pep in your step.

Skipping meals can lead to out-of-control hunger, which often results in overeating. In fact, studies show that eating regular meals is important for maintaining a healthy weight. When you're very hungry, it's very tempting (and oh-so-easy) to forget about good nutrition. Who can even *remember* the various food groups when your stomach is grumbling or when you feel light headed? Plan what you're going to eat ahead of time so you don't become confused and find yourself deliriously embracing a pint of Ben and Jerry's Cherry Garcia ice cream.

Remember earlier, when I talked about commitment and consistency? Well, you can't expect to change your way of eating overnight. As with any new habit, learning to eat healthfully takes time. In fact, you'll be more successful if you incorporate these changes into your life gradually.

It's important to think about your own food preferences and recognize the types of changes that you can make comfortably. Trying to change too much too fast can get in the way of success. Make changes one at a time and stick with them until the behaviors become a habit. The important thing is to make slow, steady, positive changes. When it comes to healthy eating, just as with exercise, you have to take it one step at a time.

HELP! I *Need Somebody*

If you're still not really sure what healthy eating is all about, I suggest you consult a professional nutritionist (also known as a registered dietitian or RD). A registered dietitian is trained to help you figure out what kind of weight loss system will mesh with your personality and lifestyle. To locate an RD in your area, ask your physician (or call the consumer nutrition hotline number listed in the Resources section at the end of this book).

9

What's Cookin' with Donna?

I'll be the first to admit that cooking is not a love of mine, but it is for my honey. Cooking in the Richardson/Sexton household is Michael's area of expertise (but you know, child, he does need my input for those final, flava-ful touches. I usually hang around to supervise). When I *do* get down in the kitchen, I have a few favorite recipes that I love to make (and eat) and want to share with you.

Mmm . . . What's Cooking?

One easy way to cut down your fat intake is to eat home-baked goods and home-prepared meals more often so that you can control the amount and types of fat that you eat. If you're too busy to cook during the week, try making big batches of soups, stews, and other foods on the weekend that you can freeze or refrigerate and reheat for later meals. (You can do this with my fruit salad, too!)

Shake It Up, Shake It Down Fruit Shake

This shake is great for breakfast, or as a preworkout pick-me-up. (Just make sure to drink it at least thirty minutes before you exercise.)

You'll need :

> 1 *cup low-fat vanilla yogurt*
> 1 *cup fresh berries*
> 1 *medium banana*
> 4 *ice cubes*

To prepare:

Put all ingredients in a blender and puree until smooth and frothy. Drink to your health! (*Makes 1 serving.*)

NUTRITION INFO PER SERVING:
387 calories; 14 g protein; 79 g carbohydrates; 3 g fat.

Fruit Olé

Fruit salad makes a wonderful addition to any breakfast, and it's great for snacks or dessert. Fresh fruit is always preferable, but you can use canned if you like. You can even combine it with low-fat yogurt or cottage cheese for a tasty, low-cal lunch.

You'll need:

> 1 *cup apples*
> *Juice of one lemon and one lime*
> 4 *cups melon*
> 2 *cups watermelon*
> 1 *cup strawberries*
> 1 *cup kiwi*
> 1 *cup blueberries*
> 1 *cup grapefruit or orange*
> 1 *cup grapes*
> 1 *cup pineapple*
> 1 *cup cherries (optional)*
> 1 *cup orange or pineapple juice*

To prepare:

Mix the apples and the lemon and lime juice together first in a large bowl (the citrus juice helps keep the apples crisp and white). Then add the remaining fruit and the orange/pineapple juice and mix well. Cover tightly and refrigerate at least two hours. Makes fourteen one-cup servings. Stir before serving. Will keep for up to one week in the fridge.

NUTRITION INFO PER SERVING:
70 calories; 1 g protein; 18 g carbohydrates; 0.5 g fat.

Donna's Delicious Pita Pocket Sandwich

Sometimes whipping up a meal can be really fun; other times it's just a chore. For those days when you'd rather be anywhere but in the kitchen, may I suggest my "short-order cook" meal. It's easy to make and even easier to eat!

You'll need:

One pita pocket per person

Leftover chicken, turkey, seafood, or steak

Lettuce and tomato or leftover vegetables

Low-fat or fat-free salad dressing of your choice

To prepare:

Simply cut open the pita, stuff in the meat and veggies (you can eat them cold or reheat them in the microwave), season to taste with the salad dressing, and *voilà*! you've got a tasty, healthy meal in under five minutes. Who said eating well had to be hard work?

NUTRITIONAL INFO PER SERVING (WITH CHICKEN OR TURKEY):
355 calories; 37 g protein; 44 g carbohydrates; 5 g fat.

WITH SEAFOOD:
305 calories; 27 g protein; 44 g carbohydrates; 2 g fat.

WITH STEAK::
448 calories; 35 g protein; 44 g carbohydrates; 16 g fat.

Miss Donna's Presto Pizza

Here's a quick, healthy recipe that kids love to make—
and eat. I often make this with my niece, cousins, and
the kids that I work with, and it's *always* a hit. (Grown-
ups love it, too!)

You'll need:

1 English muffin per person, sliced

1 jar of your favorite tomato sauce

1 package of low fat mozzarella, grated

Sliced mushrooms, onions, peppers (optional)

*A dash of oregano, garlic powder, onion powder,
basil (optional)*

To prepare:

Toast the English muffin slices lightly (until bottoms are slightly firm),
then lay them on an ungreased cookie sheet. Spoon enough sauce
onto each muffin to cover the bottom, sprinkle with the cheese, and (if
desired) add spices and vegetables. Bake at 350 degrees* for about ten
minutes (or until the cheese has melted).

NUTRITION INFO PER SERVING:
262 calories; 11 g protein; 11 g carbohydrates; 5 g fat.

*NOTE: Young children should never be left unsupervised while you
are making this recipe, and they shouldn't be allowed to go anywhere
near a hot oven. Parents or caregivers should put the pizzas into the
oven—and remove them once they are cooked—to ensure the safety of
their charges.

Quick-Fix Dinner Salad

This is one of the easiest recipes I've ever made, and it's great year-round. If you're trying to cut back on fat, make this a once-a-week staple. It's a tasty meatless meal—plus, the potatoes and asparagus make it filling.

You'll need:

4 small red new potatoes per person

3 asparagus spears per person

2 cups mixed salad greens per person

3 slices of tomato or 3 cherry tomatoes per person

2 tablespoons fat-free salad dressing

To prepare:

Put potatoes in a pot, cover with water, and bring to a boil. Simmer ten to fifteen minutes or until they're easily pierced with fork. At the same time, place asparagus in a large saucepan, cover with water, and simmer gently for two to three minutes until the stalks are tender. Meanwhile, arrange greens and tomatoes on plates. Cut the cooked potatoes in half, cut the asparagus into one-inch pieces, and add them to each plate. Serve with the fat-free dressing of your choice on the side. *Bon appetit!*

NUTRITION INFO PER SERVING:
300 calories; 9 g protein; 38 g carbohydrates; 0 g fat.

Miss D's Beer-Boiled Shrimp

This is one of my favorite lowfat recipes. In fact, it's so good that you'll probably want to make extra to have as leftovers the next day (nothing beats chilled shrimp with cocktail sauce—yum!).

You'll need:

> 1 to 2 cans beer (just enough to cover shrimp in pan)
>
> 1/2 pound of medium shrimp per person, cleaned, shelled, and deveined
>
> 1 bay leaf
>
> A generous dash of dill weed, parsley, basil, onion powder, garlic powder, and red (cayenne) pepper
>
> 3 whole peppercorns or coarse ground pepper to taste

To prepare:

Pour one can of beer into a medium-size frying pan and mix in spices and peppercorns. Add shrimp (pour in more beer if the liquid doesn't cover the shrimp), then bring the beer to a boil. As soon as beer begins boiling, remove the pan from heat. Cover and let it sit for about five minutes or until all the shrimp are bright pink and cooked through (you may have to turn some of them over). Discard liquid before serving. Serve shrimp with cocktail sauce, rice, and the vegetable of your choice (steamed zucchini with onions works nicely).

NUTRITION INFO PER SERVING (FOR BEER-BOILED SHRIMP): 120 calories; 23 g protein; 0 g carbohydrates; 2 g fat.

NUTRITION INFO PER SERVING (FOR 1 CUP RICE; 1/4 CUP COCKTAIL SAUCE, AND 1 CUP STEAMED ONIONS AND ZUCCHINI): 363 calories; 5.1 g protein; 73 g carbohydrates; 0.2 g fat.

Michael's Low-fat Eggplant Parmigiana

The trick to making this dish healthy is to use low-fat cheese and to bake, rather than fry, the eggplant slices. You get all of the taste with none of the heart-clogging grease. This is a great meal to make on the weekend and reheat during your busy work week. (Because the eggplant isn't fried and soggy, it reheats very well.) *Mangia!*

You'll need:

2 eggs

1 cup skim milk

1 cup bread crumbs (Italian seasoning optional)

3 medium eggplants, sliced in rounds $^1/4$" to $^1/2$" inch thick

2 26-ounce jars tomato sauce

1 pound low-fat mozzarella, chopped or grated

$^1/4$ cup grated Parmesan

To prepare:

Combine the eggs and milk in a shallow bowl, and put the bread crumbs in a separate bowl. Dip each slice of eggplant in the egg/milk mixture, then coat with the bread crumbs. Make sure each slice is thoroughly coated.

Spray a large baking tin with nonstick cooking spray, and arrange the eggplant slices in a single layer. Cook in a 400-degree oven for fifteen minutes or until they're tender and brown, turning once.

Put a thin layer of sauce in the bottom of a 9-by-13-inch baking dish, then add a layer of eggplant, enough sauce to cover the eggplant slices, and $^1/4$ cup of the mozzarella. Repeat this layering (eggplant, sauce, mozzarella) until you reach the last layer of eggplant. Sprinkle a generous amount of mozzarella and the Parmesan on the eggplant, then bake, uncovered, at 400 degrees for thirty minutes.

Remove from oven, and let it cool for ten to fifteen minutes before slicing. Makes ten generous servings.

> NUTRITION INFO PER SERVING:
> 146 calories; 10 g protein; 13 g carbohydrates; 5 g fat.

Big Al's Oatmeal Raisin Drop Cookies

This recipe was given to me by Dallas chef Big Al Torrence. Big Al prepares food for the syndicated radio personality Tom Joyner, a self-proclaimed cookie addict. Believe me, if Big Al was able to get my friend Tom to substitute these for the fat-filled cookies he was used to, they've *got* to be terrific. Take it from Miss D, these cookies are so good, they'll make you want to slap Mrs. Fields!

You'll need:

6 ounces light margarine (make sure it's the kind you can bake with)

1 cup brown sugar

2 eggs

1 1/2 teaspoons vanilla

7 ounces rolled oats, quick, uncooked

1 cup all purpose flour

2 teaspoons baking powder

1 teaspoon salt

1 teaspoon baking soda

1/3 cup 1% milk

3/4 cup raisins

To prepare:

Preheat oven to 375 degrees. Mix dry ingredients (flour, baking powder, salt, baking soda) together in a small bowl and set aside. Using an electric mixer, cream margarine and sugar in a mixing bowl for five minutes. Add eggs and vanilla. Continue to cream until well mixed. Add oats. Mix on low speed to blend. Alternately, add dry ingredients and milk, mixing on low speed after each addition to blend. Add raisins and stir them in by hand. Drop batter onto greased baking sheet(s), using a large spoon. Bake for twelve to fifteen minutes. Makes about three dozen cookies.

NUTRITION INFO PER SERVING (ONE SERVING EQUALS TWO COOKIES):
154 calories; 0 g protein; 0 g carbohyrates; 5 g fat.

Make It Healthy!

The way you prepare food can make a big difference in the total fat, saturated fat, and cholesterol content of a meal. Here are a few tips to make your meals even healthier:

◆ When shopping for meat, remember that certain cuts of beef and pork are leaner than others. Look for the words *round* or *loin* in the name when shopping for beef, and the words *loin* or *leg* when buying pork. When it comes to the different grades of beef, USDA "Select" beef contains the least amount of marbling (the flecks of fat within the muscle). The second leanest grade of meat is "Choice." Pork isn't graded this way, so just look for the cuts with the smallest amount of visible fat.

◆ Know what you're eating. Protein, for instance, can vary wildly when it comes to caloric make-up. Here's how the following foods can vary in their calorie content (per ounce):

> Shellfish —20 calories
>
> White meat chicken—5 to 30 calories
>
> Beef —55 to 100 calories
>
> Pork —75 to 120 calories

◆ Instead of frying, try to grill, bake, broil, or poach meat, poultry, and fish.

◆ Trim visible fat from meat and poultry before cooking. Drain additional fat after browning meat.

◆ De-fat cooked soups and stews by cooling, then skimming off the hardened fat.

◆ Steam vegetables rather than sautéing or deep-frying them.

◆ For sautéing, use nonstick pans and vegetable sprays. When basting or stir-frying, use wine, tomato juice, Worcestershire sauce, teriyaki, fruit juice, or broth instead of gravy.

◆ When you must use fats, use unsaturated vegetable oils.

◆ Use cooking techniques such as broiling or microwaving for convenience.

◆ Season with herbs and spices instead of heavy sauces.

Heart Smart Tips for Eating Out

Sometimes it's nice to let somebody else do the cooking. (I have Michael, but even he likes to have someone else do the cooking now and then, so we'll go out.) Who doesn't enjoy eating out? Someone else prepares the food, serves it, and washes the dishes afterward.

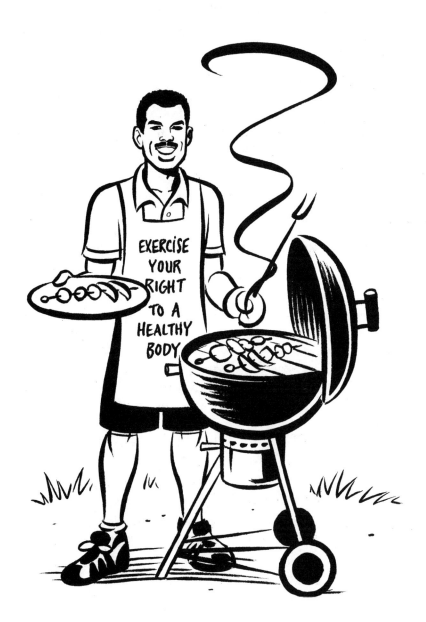

What more could you ask for? Make it a healthy, low-fat meal that doesn't make your arteries groan in protest or force you to loosen your belt a few notches. It really is possible to have your steak and eat it, too.

At Restaurants

◆ Before you eat anything, make sure to drink up—I'm talking about H_2O here, not a martini.

◆ Limit yourself to one dinner roll or a single piece of bread. You don't want to fill up before the meal arrives.

◆ Remember to ask how the food is prepared and whether substitutions can be made.

◆ Ask to have all sauces, gravy, and salad dressings served on the side. Use them sparingly, if at all.

◆ Be specific in asking for what you want. Practice these phrases: "hold the mayonnaise," "dry toast," and "dressing on the side."

◆ Order a broth-based, rather than a cream-based, soup.

◆ If you know that your entrée is going to be huge, ask the waiter to bring an extra plate, then transfer half of your meal onto the plate to take home later. (Better yet: before the entrée is even served, ask the waiter to put half of it in a doggie bag for you. What you don't see can't tempt you.)

◆ Opt for a baked potato instead of french fries.

◆ Order sorbet or fresh fruit for dessert rather than fat-and-calorie-laden confections.

Typically, a plate in a restaurant looks like this.

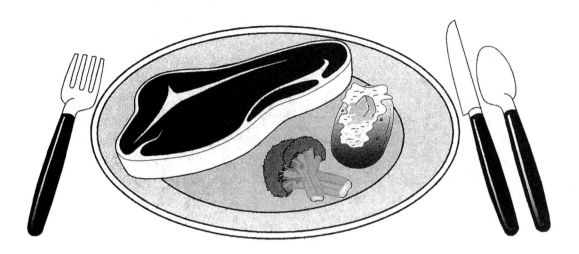

Here's what your plate *should* look like—at home or when dining out.

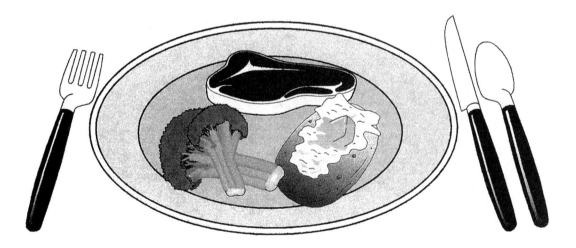

Now, I have a confession to make here. I have a special place in my heart for McDonald's, and it's not entirely because of the food (well, their french fries *are* the best). Fifteen years ago, I went into Mickey D's expecting to come out with lunch, and instead came out with a man: Michael, my honey. (I can see the headlines now: "Fitness Queen Meets Main Squeeze at Fast-Food Joint.")

I had just finished working out and had a taste for a burger and some fries. I went into the McDonald's across the street from the health club. Michael's car had broken down, and he and his college roommate were in the parking lot trying to fix it. He followed me inside and got in line behind me but couldn't think of a smooth way to introduce himself. I was oblivious to all of this and just got my order and left.

Next thing I know, I'm pulling out into three lanes of traffic, and this really cute guy is running out of McDonald's and into the middle of the street, waving his arms like a crazy man. Now that's... *not smooth.* I stopped to see what all the fuss was about, and he introduced himself and asked for my phone number. I never give my number to strangers, but I took his card and called him a few weeks later. (What can I say? I was intrigued by this guy who risked his life just to say hello.) We started dating, and the rest is history.

As you can see, fast food is not entirely a bad thing. While I can't promise you love, I can still offer some suggestions for keeping things healthy.

At Fast-Food Joints

♦ When it comes to high-fat foods, practice the "either/or" method of calorie control: order the burger *or* the french fries; the mashed potatoes *or* the biscuit; the onion rings *or* the milkshake.

♦ Instead of ordering a pepperoni or sausage pizza, try one with mushrooms, peppers, or other vegetables.

◆ Order sandwiches on whole-wheat, pita, or rye bread instead of on high-fat croissants.

◆ Choose foods that have been grilled or broiled rather than fried.

◆ Instead of tartar sauce, mayonnaise, and other creamy sauces, opt for a little ketchup or, even better, mustard (it has less sugar).

◆ Skip the cheese and the special sauces on the burger—order a mushroom burger instead, or be daring and order a veggie or tofu burger. (Don't knock it till you try it!)

◆ Have the chicken sandwich. It's usually lower in fat and calories than any other entrée choice (including the fried fish sandwich).

◆ Use vinaigrette, low-fat, or fat-free salad dressing.

◆ Order low-fat chocolate milk instead of a milkshake. It has more calcium with a fraction of the fat and calories.

Cuisines with Flava

International restaurants are as varied as the countries they represent. Here are a few suggestions to help you make wise choices at your favorite restaurants.

Positive Choices	Diner Beware!
Italian	
Minestrone soup	Antipasto plates
Breadsticks	Buttered garlic bread
Vinegar and oil dressing	Creamy Italian dressing
Pasta with red sauce such as marinara	Creamy white, pesto, or butter sauces such as Alfredo
Chicken cacciatore	Italian sausage
Piccata or florentine	Scallopine or parmigiana
Marsala or clam sauce	Alfredo or carbonara sauce
Cappuccino	Italian ice cream
Chinese	
Wonton soup	Fried wontons
Hot and sour soup	Egg drop soup
Soft noodles	Crispy fried noodles
Steamed dumplings	Fried egg rolls
Beef with broccoli	Sweet and sour pork or shrimp
Moo Shu Pork	Lemon chicken
Chicken, scallops, or shrimp with vegetables	Egg fu young
	Peking duck
Steamed rice	Fried rice

POSITIVE CHOICES	DINER BEWARE!

Mexican

Black bean soup, menudo	Guacamole dip with taco chips
Salsa	Sour cream and cheese
Soft, plain tortillas	Crispy, fried tortillas
Burritos, soft tacos, enchiladas, tamales	Tacos, taco salad, tostadas, chile rellenos, quesadillas
Picante or mole sauce	Cheese sauce
Spicy beef	Chorizo (Mexican sausage)
Salsa verde	Refried beans

Thai

Spicy shrimp soup	Any type of coconut soup
Basil or basil sauce	Peanuts or peanut sauce
Chili or lime sauce or crushed, dried chilis	Curry sauce (usually contains coconut milk)
Thai spices	*Anything* made with coconut milk
Yum	Pad Thai
Fish sauce, hot sauce	Eggplant (it's usually fried)

Japanese

Yaki (broiled) or yakimono (grilled)	Tempura (batter-dipped and deep fried)
Teriyaki	Katsu
Miso soup	Fried tofu
Sushi or sashimi	Una ju (eel)
Nabemono	Agemono
Seasoned rice	Fried rice

Positive Choices	Diner Beware!

Indian

Mulligatawny (lentil soup)	Coconut soup
Tandoori or tikka	Kurma
Curry sauce	Coconut or almond sauce
Dal (lentils)	Ghee (clarified butter)
Naan bread	Poori bread
Masala sauce	Molee sauce (coconut)

Soul Food

Skinless chicken or turkey	Chitterlings or hog maws
Fish or lean beef	Pig feet or pig tails
Lean veal chops and roasts	Spare ribs or sausage
Center-cut ham	Ham hocks
Canadian bacon	Regular bacon
Pork tenderloin or loin chops	Oxtails or goat
Vegetables and beans prepared with skinless turkey parts and seasonings	Vegetables and beans prepared with fat back, neck bones, salt pork, ham hocks, or coconut oil.
Hominy grits with margarine	Hominy grits with butter
Baked macaroni and low-fat cheese	Baked macaroni and regular cheese
Baked or boiled potatoes	Home fries

10

An Apple a Day

Being "fit" means different things to different people. To a professional athlete, physical conditioning is the vital link to peak performance. To some gym bunnies, it means having tight buns, six-pack abs, and shapely arms. For the rest of us, it's more about meeting the demands of our everyday routines with energy and zest. The health benefits of eating well and being active are both physical and mental: a healthy lifestyle can lower your risk for many diseases, increase longevity, improve self-esteem, and boost your ability to manage stress. Who doesn't want to live longer and feel better doing it? (I do! I do!) Looking fit and fine is just an added bonus (but what a bonus it is). I always feel more energetic and upbeat after a good workout, and I definitely get fewer colds when I take the time to eat right and exercise. But adopting healthier habits can prevent things far more serious than the flu.

The 10 Leading Causes of Death in the United States

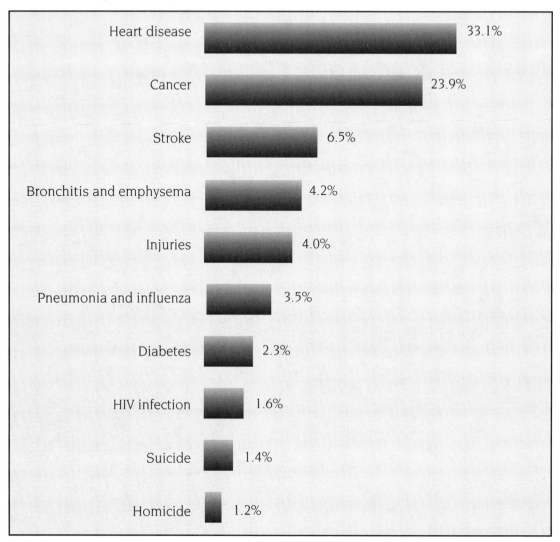

The Centers for Disease Control (CDC), the government's leading prevention agency, has identified these as the top ten causes of death. While there are certain "fixed" factors that determine whether or not you'll develop a chronic disease (such as heredity, age, and environment), six of the top ten killers can be prevented—even reversed—through simple lifestyle changes!

According to *Healthy People* 2000, a report put out by the Department of Health & Human Services, if all Americans ate fewer high-fat foods and did just thirty minutes of moderate activity each day, about 400,000 lives would be saved annually. The incidence of heart disease, stroke, cancer, and diabetes would plummet. Did you know that a sedentary lifestyle nearly <u>doubles</u> (*doubles*!!) a person's risk for heart disease, and that bad eating habits are associated with five of the ten leading causes of death in the United States? Shocking but true. Let's take a look at "the big three."

Heart Disease

The statistics on diet and heart disease are compelling. According to the American Heart Association (AHA), cardiovascular disease (a term that encompasses heart attack, stroke, rheumatic heart disease, and high blood pressure) causes 926,000 deaths in the United States each year—claiming 479,000 women and 447,000 men. This amounts to more than all cancer-related deaths combined.

Heart attacks are the single largest killer of Americans, both male and female. About every twenty seconds an American will suffer a heart attack, and about every minute someone will die from one. This year, it's estimated that as many as 1.5 million Americans will have a heart attack, and about one-third of them will die. A heart attack (also known as coronary heart disease) occurs when the supply of blood to the heart muscle is severely reduced or stopped. This happens because one (or more) of the coronary arteries that supplies blood to the heart is blocked by fat and cholesterol deposits, or by a blood clot (it's that taco deluxe coming back to haunt you—literally). Depending upon how long the blood supply is cut off, the muscle cells in that area of the heart suffer permanent damage—or die.

Heart disease is not an equal-opportunity killer: it kills more African-Americans than it does people of other races, and while men suffer more heart attacks than women, studies show that 44 percent of women die within a year of having a heart attack, as compared to 27 percent of men. And in about 48 percent of men and 63 percent of women who died suddenly of a heart attack, there was no previous evidence of disease. Frightening, isn't it? My grandmother, who was sitting at her usual spot at the dining room table, cutting up vegetables, had a heart attack. She died before they could get her to the hospital.

Fortunately, heart disease is easily preventable through a sensible eating and exercise program. A low-fat diet inhibits the promotion of blood cholesterol, which is the main culprit in the development of atherosclerosis (the medical term for clogged arteries and blood vessels). Exercise works against heart disease by increasing the amount of oxygen drawn into the lungs, which in turn forces the heart to work more efficiently, even while at rest. It also prevents or delays the development of high blood pressure and reduces blood pressure in people who already have hypertension. Physical activity also helps by raising the level of HDL (or "good") cholesterol, which reduces your risk of developing blood clots and diabetes.

Cancer

In 1997, more than 560,000 people died of cancer, and almost 1.4 million new cases were diagnosed. The typical American diet, which is high in fat and calories and low in fiber, fruits, and vegetables, is definitely part of the problem. Almost half of all cancer deaths are related to what you eat. If you change what you eat, you can change your odds for getting certain types of cancer. Research suggests that the bile our bodies produce to digest high-fat foods promotes colon cancer. The nitrates found in smoked meats and foods are thought to promote cancer of the stomach and esophagus. The excess estrogen that's produced by an overweight woman's body puts her at an increased risk for breast cancer.

Unfortunately, breast cancer strikes one out of every nine women. Every three minutes a woman is diagnosed with breast cancer, and every twelve minutes the disease claims another life. Who among us doesn't know someone who has survived—or succumbed to—breast cancer?

There is hope. The National Cancer Institute estimates that significant reductions in cancer incidence could be achieved by the year 2000 if all Americans adopted the low-fat, high-fiber diet outlined in the Food Guide Pyramid, and participated in a regular moderate exercise program. In other words, you *can* prevent many types of cancer. What more incentive do you need to get up and move, and into the health groove?

Stroke

On average, someone suffers a stroke in the United States every minute, and every 3.5 minutes the disease claims a life. A stroke occurs when fat and cholesterol build up in the arteries or blood vessel walls leading to the brain. (See, what you eat *can* be hazardous to your health.) Oftentimes, a blood clot forms in the narrowed artery and blocks off the blood vessel completely, resulting in a stroke (or "brain attack") .

Even people who should know better don't always take the steps to prevent a stroke from occurring. My own father—who's been taking high blood pressure medication for the past few years—suffered a second stroke in 1994. I've been trying to get him to quit smoking and to eat right and exercise for as long as I can remember. I'll keep on trying until he makes his health a top priority.

If you make healthy habits an ongoing part of your life, you're practicing preventative medicine. Prevention really is the best medicine, and the good news is that it's never too late to adopt these life-enhancing behaviors.

A while back my mom lost thirty-five pounds after many years of being unhappy with the way she looked and felt. I had tried to motivate her for a *looong* time, but she just wasn't ready to hear it. You know how parents always say their kids don't listen? Well, there was a complete role reversal here. Mom was so busy taking care of other people that she wasn't taking care of herself. (How many of you can relate to that scenario? Are you feeling a sense of déjà vu?) Her busy schedule left her exhausted (she rarely ate dinner before ten at night), with low self-esteem, a serious weight problem, and a couple of unattended health problems (not to mention the fact that she had less kick in her step on the dance floor). She would do her signature move—shaking her groove thang down to the floor—but she started having trouble getting her groove thang back up again. My mom *loooves* to dance, and you can imagine how it feels when you can't do what you love.

For years, I had been trying to show her how to incorporate good nutrition and daily exercise into her life. The information fell on deaf ears. She took diet pills, ate one meal a day, exercised sporadically, and would take laxatives and drink teas to try to lose weight. All this taught me one thing: you can't help someone until they're ready to help themselves.

One day right after Mom retired, she came to me, and said, "I'm ready for this now. I'm tired of being overweight, I'm tired of not having energy. The other day, I had to buy a new dress for a church function, and I couldn't fit into a size twelve anymore. I couldn't even fit into a fourteen! By the time I tried on a size sixteen—which fit—I was almost crying. Donna, I've made up my mind and I'm ready to make a change."

Mom began slowly. I helped her by designing a workout program that included activities she enjoyed. She began walking regularly and started using my exercise videos several times a week. I also got her to do a stretching program, along with strength training (her least favorite part of the workout). She walked and stretched on Wednesdays and Fridays, did aerobics and strength training on Mondays and Thursdays, and went out dancing on the weekends. Within nine months, she lost thirty-five pounds—and had energy to burn.

Of course, it wasn't always easy going—at the start, she found the program really challenging. I made sure that no matter what city or country I was in, I gave my mom a pep call to offer her encouragement and support. If I wasn't calling her, she was calling me: to complain that she didn't have a new videotape to work out with, or that she didn't have anyone to walk with. Other times, she'd call to toot her horn about how good she felt and looked.

I also worked with my mom to change her eating habits. I encouraged her to cut down on fatty foods and increase the amount of fruits and vegetables she ate. She was notorious for eating fried foods late into the night, snacking on junk food, skipping meals, and attending a fish fry at my grandmother's house every Friday evening. (Now I do enjoy my fried fish, fried potatoes, buttery cabbage, and cornbread—in moderation. The *m* word was something Mom had to learn.) She slowly adopted a healthier menu and learned to prepare foods in a healthier way. She had a few setbacks—"Drop that drumstick, Mom!"—but she met those challenges and kept marching forward.

Today, almost four years later, she's hittin' and holdin'. She's kept the weight off and continues to eat well and exercise at least three times a week. We often power walk or work out with one of my videos together, which I love because it gives us a chance to talk and just spend time with each other. Now she's as bad as she wants to be (I mean that in a good way), and she out-boogies *me* on the dance floor. She's a great role model for anybody who's trying to get into better shape, and I'm really proud of her accomplishment. It took time and effort, but she did it. (In fact, she now leads her own exercise class in the church basement. I mean what's next? LaVerne's workout tape?!) Seriously, I have three words for you, Mom: *You go, girl!*

Even when you've made a commitment to healthy living, using healthy habits as preventative medicine is sometimes easier said than done—even within my own family. During the course of my career as a fitness professional, I've been preaching the benefits of healthy eating and physical activity to my relatives as well as my clients. With my family though, my advice usually went in one ear and out the other. But when several of my older family members got sick, and were advised by their physicians to take better care of themselves, my words suddenly started to sink in. "You mean I could have been doing this all along and then I wouldn't have gotten ill?" they asked me. Yup. Even my teenage niece, Tara, who used to ignore her health, now works out twice a week with her favorite Auntie's video and plays basketball. These days I'm the resident fitness expert: "Donna, what kind of walking shoes should I buy?" "Donna, how often do I need to exercise to lower my high blood pressure?" "Donna, have you got any tips for making macaroni and cheese without all the fat?"

Now, I'm sorry that it took an illness to make some of my relatives rethink their old habits, but I'm thrilled that they've finally seen the light—and that I can be there to help guide them through the sometimes confusing world of food and fitness. I'm here to guide *you* through that world, too.

Weight management is vital to maintaining good health, preventing disease, and in enhancing the quality of your life. The key is to determine what weight is best for you, then maintain it by eating well-balanced meals and staying active.

Managing your weight, like managing anything else, takes some time and effort. Here are some tips that work for me and my clients:

1. *Think long-term, act gradually.* It's true that fasting and starvation-type diets can peel off pounds quickly, and grueling exercise regimens can't help but tone the body. But they are short-term solutions to a lifetime concern. Instead of trying quick fixes, gradually make realistic changes in your lifestyle. Try one new low-fat meal per week. Begin taking a fifteen- or twenty-minute walk every other morning.

2. *Stick to a schedule.* There is no hard and fast rule about eating three square meals a day; nevertheless, it does help to establish regular eating habits. Missed meals can lead to impulsive snacking and overeating and can even lower the rate at which your body burns calories. People who eat three meals a day plus two snacks lose weight more easily than those who eat only one big meal a day.

3. *Variety is the spice of life.* It's also the key to successful weight loss. Have a protein in combination with a carbohydrate at breakfast, lunch, and dinner. In fact, it's a good idea to have something from as many of the food groups as possible at each meal. This is also true of exercise. Mix it up to keep it fun (cross-training is the secret of my success)!

4. *Enlist support.* Having family and friends join you in your efforts to trim the fat and keep active certainly increases the enjoyment factor; it also gives you support that can help keep your efforts on track. Those who have the support of family members, particularly the support of their spouses, are more likely to manage their weight successfully.

5. *Cut yourself some slack.* Nobody's perfect. Allow for occasional slipups and indulgences. Food and exercise are both meant to be enjoyed. If you eat cheesecake at lunch, relish the splurge. Then balance that higher-fat indulgence with a low-fat dinner of broiled fish and steamed vegetables. Don't use one slipup as an excuse to give up. Get back on

track at the very next meal. Successful weight control is not measured by a number on the scale or a too-strict lifestyle. It comes from knowing that you are eating and exercising in ways that make a positive contribution to your health.

6. *There are no "good" or "bad" foods.* Any food can fit into a healthy way of eating. The key is to balance your choices over time so that your overall diet is sound. If you want to indulge in a favorite food that may be high in fat and sugar, just moderate your portion size and how often you eat it. Buy a small bag of pretzels or chips, for example, rather than tempting yourself with the jumbo size. Take three cookies out of the box and savor them slowly rather than mindlessly devouring the entire package. When eating out, split a high-fat entrée with your dining companion, or order an appetizer-size portion of your favorite high-fat food, rounding out the meal with a salad, vegetables, and a starch.

7. *Add, rather than eliminate, foods.* To fill up while still cutting back on portions at a meal, add hot or cold vegetable juice, broth, clear consommé, salad, raw vegetables, or fruit as an appetizer. If you're eating a late dinner out, have a piece of fruit before going to the restaurant so that you don't attack the bread basket or order unwisely.

8. *Be prepared.* The Boy Scouts have the right idea. *Always* keep healthy foods at home. Ideally, you should have fresh food on hand. But sometimes it just doesn't work out that way. If you can't get to the supermarket more than once a week, stock up. Every healthy pantry should contain: frozen and canned fruits and veggies, small cans of water-packed fish (tuna, salmon, sardines), low-fat soups, dry and cooked cereal, frozen meats in moderate-size portions (three-ounce turkey patties and skinless chicken cutlets), dairy snacks (such as fat-free pudding and yogurt), Parmalat 1% or skim milk. Pretzels and air-popped popcorn make healthy snacks. This way, you'll always have healthy, low-fat foods on hand that are ready-to-eat or quick to prepare.

9. *Preparation is also key when it comes to staying fit.* Stash a pair of sneakers in your trunk or office and take a walk at lunch or during a coffee break.

Schedule workouts into your calendar so you won't be tempted to skip them. Instead of meeting a friend for dinner, why not meet for a mall walk (stroll while you window shop), or hook up for a bike ride on the weekend. Make fitness an integral part of your everyday life.

10. A *healthy mind makes for a healthy body*. One way to de-stress and keep your mind sharp is to try meditating, deep breathing, reading a good book, listening to your favorite music, playing a game of chess or backgammon—or do like I do and put on your dancing shoes and dance the night away (I *loove* that Latin beat).

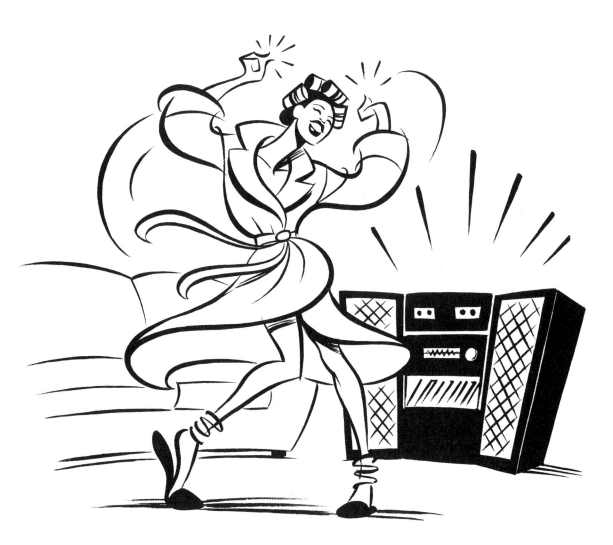

11

Let's Get Real!

Y ou now have the keys to healthy living right in the palm of your hand. The main key to improving yourself—mentally and physically—is by learning self-acceptance. Once you feel good about yourself, you'll see how important it is to make your health and well-being a priority.

Remember: getting fit will take time and effort. But you're worth it, right? Feeling good about yourself also allows you to feel good about others. We often get so caught up in the day-to-day grind that we forget to look outward. We need to look beyond ourselves and help other people. One of my greatest pleasures is helping people (like you) reach their full potential. My goal in writing this book is to help you get fit and stay fit. I've given you the tips and tools you need to get started, but the rest is up to you.

Several years ago, my best friend and colleague Charles Little and I were walking around downtown D.C. Out of nowhere, this young woman came up to me and said, "Excuse me. You have my body. God obviously made a mistake and gave you my body, and I got stuck with this one." (She wasn't fat, but she wasn't in the best of shape, either.)

I was flattered at the compliment, but it left me speechless. Charles, never at a loss for words, jumped right in. "Child, put down those cheese fries and then we can talk." She ignored him and continued talking to me.

"I know you're in fitness. Can you help me get the body I was supposed to have? Tina Turner's legs, Madonna's arms, and your abs."

As ridiculous as her request was, it's not at all uncommon. A lot of people think the only way they can look great is to look like somebody else. But you shouldn't want to look like someone else—you should be thankful for what you have and start working on becoming a better you.

This advice applies to everyone. No amount of dieting and exercise is going to make you look like Tina, Madonna—or even me. What good nutrition and regular physical activity can do, however, is help improve what God gave you. There's only one you in this world, and I'm here to help you make the most of it.

Oftentimes, beginning an exercise program is the simple part—the hard part is sticking with it. It's so easy to get tempted when you can barely go a mile without seeing those golden arches or a big chicken bucket looming in the sky. J. Anthony Brown, a colleague of mine from the *Tom Joyner Morning Show*, had recently started my GetFit Walking Program when he ran into trouble. One morning he told me how he had been out walking the day before when he heard the voice of the Colonel calling his name. He succumbed to the pressure, and before he knew it he was continuing his walk with a water bottle in one hand and a two-piece fried chicken dinner with mashed potatoes, gravy, and biscuits in the other. Since I am the resident fitness expert on Tom's show, I came up with a special walk/run program tailored for J. Anthony and people like him: walk until you get to the Colonel's house, then turn around and run like hell!

Seriously, though, you have to expect a few setbacks as you venture down the road to wellness. Sometimes the path will be clear, other times you may have to jump over a few obstacles (Häagen-Dazs and Krispy Kreme Donuts always get *me* a little sidetracked). The point is, you may fall off the wagon, but don't let the wagon drag you along. You have to get back on track and keep moving in the right direction.

A technique that I use to help me achieve my goals is visualization. I mentally envision—in exact detail—what it is I want to achieve, and then I map out a plan as to how I'm going to make it a reality. Professional athletes often use this technique to put themselves in a winning frame of mind, but it can be applied to pretty much any situation in life. You can picture yourself crossing the finish line of a marathon, obliterating your tennis opponent, fitting into that sexy

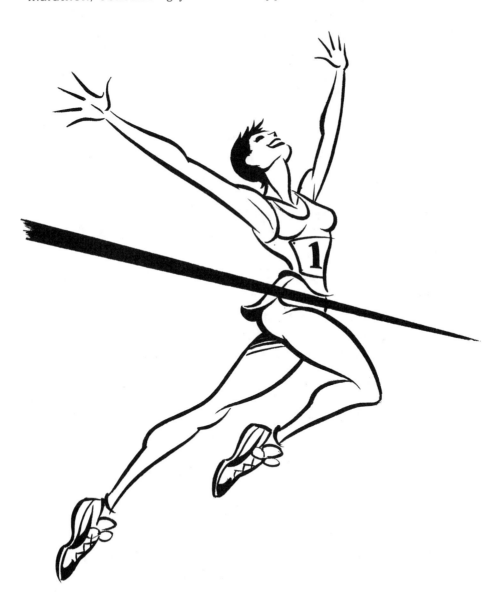

party dress, or sitting in the boardroom chairing a meeting. Once you've visualized what it is you want to accomplish, sit down and figure out exactly what you have to do to make it happen (jot down notes if it helps). Whatever your goal is, I really believe that if you live it mentally, you can achieve it physically. The key is to formulate a workable game plan to make those dreams a reality.

And (*mucho importante*) don't forget to congratulate yourself on everything that you achieve—no matter how ."small" that victory may seem. After all, it takes just as much effort not to give up during a tough workout as it does to land a big account at work. Take time to honor yourself and to celebrate your accomplishments—large and small—each and every day. The more you come to view yourself in a positive light, the easier it becomes to take care of yourself and to make your health and well-being a top priority. (It's too easy to give up if you don't feel deserving.) Focus on the positive feelings that eating well and exercising bring you. Rejoice in your newfound inner strength, energy, confidence, and lifestyle. When it comes to bodies, there is only one per customer. Changing old habits may take some time and effort, but (to paraphrase that infamous hair color ad): "You're worth it."

As I often tell my clients, the only disability is a bad attitude. Think of yourself as "the little engine that could." It may sound trite, but I assure you, it's true: if you think you can, you can. And if you think you can't, you're right! So repeat after me: "I think I can, I think I can, I think I can, I think I can." Actually, a better mantra might be: "I *know* I can." You've come this far, right?! So what's stopping you from going the distance and achieving your all-time personal best? *Nothing*, that's what. You just need to get out of your own way—no negative self-talk, no "all or nothing" ultimatums, no unrealistic ("I'm gonna drop ten pounds in five days!") goals—and take it one day at a time. The real key to success—whether it's getting fit, reaching the top of your profession, or a having a good relationship—is determination and stick-to-it-iveness. Think "I will" not "I should." Remember what I said at the beginning of this book? *Good health is not a destination, it's a journey.* So hop in, buckle up, and enjoy the ride!

All the tools you need to stay the course are right here in this book. Miss Donna has broken it down and given you the real deal. Despite what those infomercials may tell you, there aren't any easy answers. The secret to healthy living isn't so secret, after all (and it doesn't come in a box for three easy payments of $29.95). Incorporate some of the tips I've given you into your daily life, and you'll be well on your way to a better future—mentally, physically, and spiritually. Take it one step at a time, and soon these healthy habits will become second nature. Are we seeing eye-to-eye? Are you clear about Miss Donna's Basics? Alright, then. *Let's Get Real!* It's time to exercise your right to a healthy body.

Fitness/Nutrition Log

Day	1	2	3
Breakfast			
Mid-Morning Snack			
Lunch			
Mid-Afternoon Snack			
Supper			
Evening Snack/ Dessert			
Exercise			
Wellness			

4	5	6	7

Sample Log

Day	Monday	Tuesday	Wednesday
Breakfast	Coffee w/skim milk 1 cup LF yogurt 1 banana 1 cup o.j.	Coffee w/skim milk 8 oz. Shake It Up, Shake It Down Fruit Shake (w/strawber- ries and blueberries)	Coffee w/skim milk 1 cup raisin bran w/1 cup skim milk 1/2 melon 1 cup o.j.
Mid-Morning Snack	none	1 plum	none
Lunch	Pita Pocket Sand- wich w/3 oz. chicken breast, lettuce, tomato, onion, 2 tbsp. honey mustard	3 oz. roast beef on a roll w/lettuce, toma- to & LF mayo	4 oz. turkey on whole wheat w/LF mayo, tomato, let- tuce, onion, sprouts 8 oz. apple juice
Mid-Afternoon Snack	1 cup Fruit Olé fruit salad	4 oz. leftover fruit shake	none
Supper	3 oz. grilled salmon w/1 cup boiled new potatoes and 1 cup steamed broccoli 2 cups salad w/LF dressing	3 cups Quick-Fix Salad w/FF dressing and 2 oz. cheese 1 plain roll	2 cups rice w/1 cup black beans (made w/garlic, onions, cilantro) (Yum!)
Evening Snack/ Dessert	1 cup LF frozen yogurt	none	1 cup FF pudding
Exercise	Walked 45 minutes, did crunches and stretches	Strength training, 20-minute bike ride, stretches	Walked 45 min., did crunches and stretches
Wellness	15 min. meditation in the morning	Read a chapter of "In the Spirit"	1 hr. volunteer work

Thursday	Friday	Saturday	Sunday
Coffee w/skim milk ½ cup FF cottage cheese w/pineapple 1 cup grapefruit juice 1 banana	Coffee w/ skim milk 1 cup Fruit Olé fruit salad 1 cup LF yogurt	Coffee w/skim milk 2 poached eggs 2 slices whole wheat toast 1 cup o.j.	Coffee w/skim milk 8 oz. Shake It Up, Shake It Down Fruit Shake (w/bananas and strawberries)
1 cup LF yogurt	8 oz. can tomato juice	none	none
3 cups mixed greens w/cukes, tomatoes, mushrooms, 1 oz. feta cheese, 2 tbsp. FF dressing 1 plain roll	Lunch out w/girls from work: Bowl of veggie soup 2 cups Caesar salad w/3oz. grilled chicken, dressing on the side, 1 slice of chocolate cake	1 serving Miss Donna's Presto Pizza w/the kids and Jim	2 cups Quick-Fix Salad w/2 tbsp. LF dressing
1 cup watermelon	none	none	8 oz. skim milk w/2 graham crackers
2 cups pasta w/3 2 oz. meatballs, 1 cup red sauce, 2 tbsp. Parmesan 1 slice Italian bread	1 serving Miss D's Beer-Boiled Shrimp w/1 cup wild rice 1 cup steamed zucchini and onions	6 stuffed mushrooms 6 oz. filet mignon w/1 cup garlic mashed potatoes and 1 cup spinach 2 glasses red wine	1 serving Michael's LF Eggplant w/1 slice Italian bread 1 glass red wine
Big Al's LF Oatmeal Raisin Cookies (2)	1 cup pineapple	none	none
Strength training and stretches 20 mins. on StairMaster	1 hr. kickboxing class before work	20 mins. of yoga (before the kids woke up)	Day of rest
15 min. meditation before bed	Took kids to a baseball game	Dinner & dancing w/ my honey	Church

Resources

❑

Exercise Equipment

Xertube by Spri Products, Inc.
800-222-7774, Dept. 77

Call to order the Xertube workout band (featured in the *Let's Get Real!* travel program in chapter 4). The band comes in four different color-coded resistances (from least difficult to hardest): Yellow ($3.75), Green ($4), Red ($5), and Blue ($6). Spri also makes the Xerbar ($29), which can be used in conjunction with the Xertube to do strength-training and balance-enhancing exercises.

Donna's Products

Donna Richardson's videotapes are available through:

Anchor Bay Entertainment, Inc.
800-910-7766, extension 242

Call to order any of Donna's videos, including 30-Days to Thinner Thighs, 30-Days to Firmer Abs and Arms, Donna-Mite Aerobics, 4-Day Rotation Workout, Step & Awesome Abs, Back to Basics ($14.98 each) or Attitude Aerobics ($9.99).

To order Donna's "Donnamite" workout audiocassettes ($12.95) or her "Exercise Your Right to a Healthy Body" T-shirt ($14.95), call 800-882-0291. (A portion of the proceeds from T-shirt sales will help fund Donna's StayFit Kids program.)

To order Donna-endorsed Spa Chic products (Boost Workout Lotion, Freshen-Up Body Lotion, Magic Bath Drops, or Stress-Relief Massage Oil, $9.95 for each 4-ounce bottle), call 800-749-5713.

Visit Donna online at: http://www.tjms.com

Exercise Info

The exercise chapters of *Let's Get Real!* were researched and written with the help of Tim Moore, Ph.D. Tim is an exercise physiologist in Southern California and a fitness editor at *Shape* magazine.

American Council on Exercise (ACE)
800-825-3636
Internet address: http://www.acefitness.org

Call or log on to receive free ACE Fit Fact info sheets.

President's Council on Physical Fitness and Sports
202-690-6900

Call for free pamphlets and brochures (including the kid's workout booklet "Get Fit!: A Handbook for Youth Ages 6–17").

American College of Sports Medicine (ACSM)
P. O. Box 1440
Indianapolis, IN 46206
Internet address: http://www.acsm.org/sportsmed

Send a SASE (self-addressed, stamped envelope) to receive ACSM's general information brochure.

Disease Prevention Information

American Heart Association
800-AHA-USA1

Call for free brochures on preventing heart disease and stroke.

American Cancer Society
800-ACS-2345

Call for free brochures on cancer prevention.

American Institute for Cancer Research

800-843-8114

Call for free pamphlets on cancer prevention.

Cancer Information Service

800-4-CANCER

Ask for the free booklet "Action Guide for Healthy Eating."

CDC National AIDS Clearinghouse

800-458-5231

Ask for the free booklet "Caring for Someone with AIDS at Home" and the "Eating Defensively" brochure.

Exercise for Older Adults

President's Council on Physical Fitness and Sports

202-690-6900

Ask for the free booklet "Pep Up Your Life: A Fitness Book for Mid-Life and Older Persons."

Kids' Organizations

Nike's P.L.A.Y. Program (Participate in the Lives of America's Youth)

800-929-PLAY

Call for more info on how to get involved in keeping kids active.

Boys & Girls Club of America

800-854-CLUB

Call for info on how to get involved in your area.

Big Brothers/Big Sisters of America

215-567-7000

Call for more info on how to get involved in your area.

YWCA

800-YWCA-US1, extension 7960

Call to learn how to get involved in your area.

Nutrition Information

The nutrition chapters of *Let's Get Real!* were researched and written with the help of Lorraine Eyerman, M.A., R.D., a nutritionist in New York City. In addition to her private practice, Lorraine is a nutrition consultant to the American Heart Association; the American Dietetic Association; and SHARE, a breast cancer support group.

American Dietic Association (ADA)
800-366-1566

Call for free brochures on healthy eating (for adults and children), or to find a registered dietitian/nutritionist in your area. You can also access the ADA online at: http://www.eatright.org

If you don't need to make a personal appointment with an R.D., but do have nutrition questions you'd like answered, you can call 900-225-5267 to speak with an ADA-certified nutritionist (at a cost of $1.95 for the first minute, 95 cents thereafter; an average call lasts four minutes).

International Food Information Council site
Internet address: http://ificinfo.health.org/

The IFIC's website provides all sorts of nutrition and food safety info, and you can also use it to order free brochures and pamphlets.

University of Illinois Nutrition Analysis Tool site
Internet address: http://www.ag.uiuc.edu/~food~lab/nat/

You list what you've eaten, and the program calculates your caloric, protein, fat, calcium, iron, and vitamin intake, and tells you if you're not getting enough of certain nutrients and how to get them.

Eating Disorders Information

ANAD (the National Association of Anorexia Nervosa and Associated Disorders)
P. O. Box 7
Highland Park, IL 60035
847-831-3438

Call for free literature or to be referred to a therapist in your area.

American Anorexia/Bulimia Association
165 West 46th Street, suite 1108
New York, New York 10036
212-575-6200

Call for free literature or professional referrals.

International Association of Eating Disorders Professionals
123 NW 13th Street, suite 206
Boca Raton, FL 33432
561-338-6494

Call for a referral to an eating disorders therapist in your area.

Additional Reading

In the Spirit: The Inspirational Writings of Susan L. Taylor (Harper Perennial, 1994).

The Six Pillars of Self-Esteem by Nathaniel Branden (Bantam, 1995).

Put your fitness plans in fast forward.

You've read Donna's book, now choose from a variety of her award-winning fitness videos!

Order today! Call 1-800-910-7766, ext. 242

NEW!

30 Days to Thinner Thighs   45 min. $14.98
Thinner, firmer hips and thighs are achievable in just 30 days with these calorie-burning aerobics and concentrated toning exercises.

NEW!

30 Days to Firmer Abs & Arms   45 min. $14.98
Sleek, toned abs and arms are possible in 30 days by combining highly-effective toning exercises with calorie-burning aerobics in a workout that is fun to do.

4 Day Rotation Workout   60 min. $14.98
Excellent rating from Consumer's Report. Choose one of four 15 minute programs each day, and you'll strengthen and tone your entire body.

Donna-Mite Aerobic Workout   53 min. $14.98
5-Star Review from Fitness Magazine. This mixed impact aerobic workout is easy to follow, fun and has great music!

Back To Basics   65 min. $14.98
On Woman's Day "10 Workout Videos That Deliver" list. A common-sense approach to fitness and weight maintenance.

Step and Awesome Abs   60 min. $14.98
Rated Best Step Aerobics by SELF Magazine. A tightening, toning and stamina-building workout.

Attitude Aerobics   39 min. $9.99
A low impact, high energy workout filled with fun and funky moves.

500 Kirts Boulevard,
Troy, MI 48084
Distributed by Anchor Bay Entertainment
© 1998 Anchor Bay Entertainment